Allergies, Poisoning and Intolerance to Common Substances

Marlon Gustavo Múnera Gómez
Oscar Correa Jimenez • Juana Bustillo Arias
Editors

Allergies, Poisoning and Intolerance to Common Substances

Basic and Clinical Aspects

Springer

Editors
Marlon Gustavo Múnera Gómez
Faculty of Health
Corporación Universitaria Rafael Nuñez
Cartagena, Colombia

Oscar Correa Jimenez
Department of Pediatrics
Universidad Nacional de Colombia
Bogotá, Colombia

Juana Bustillo Arias
Neuroimmune SAS Medical
Monteria, Colombia

ISBN 978-3-031-93657-9 ISBN 978-3-031-93658-6 (eBook)
https://doi.org/10.1007/978-3-031-93658-6

This Springer imprint is published by the registered company Springer Nature Switzerland AG
The registered company address is: Gewerbestrasse 11, 6330 Cham, Switzerland

I dedicate this book to all the curious minds who are not satisfied with what is taken for granted. Those who seek to quench their thirst for knowledge in the classroom, in books, and through their mentors. To those minds that do not conform to preset schedules, that ask uncomfortable questions because there is always more to learn. To them, this book—born from children of public education—because learning is also a political act, as it allows us to envision a different world.

To the girl in red, C.A., because this book was also made possible by the strength of her love and trust in me.

To Tomás, so that in the future he may witness the work of his father, Emiro, who was not only an excellent professional and father but also a great friend. Thank you for standing firm to see this great project through to completion.

Preface

Allergies, poisoning, and intolerance represent complex interactions between environmental exposures and the human immune system, often leading to significant clinical and public health challenges. Understanding these interactions at both the basic and clinical levels is essential for developing effective diagnostic tools, preventive strategies, and therapeutic interventions.

This book, *Basic and Clinical Aspects of Allergies, Poisoning, and Intolerance*, provides a comprehensive and multidisciplinary exploration of these conditions, offering valuable insights into their mechanisms, manifestations, and management. The content is designed to bridge the gap between fundamental research and clinical practice, facilitating a deeper understanding of how various biological agents, chemicals, and foods impact human health.

Each chapter is authored by experts in the fields of immunology, toxicology, pharmacology, and clinical medicine. The book covers a diverse range of topics, including the allergenicity and toxicological aspects of *Cannabis sativa*, the parasitic and allergic implications of *Anisakis simplex*, and the mechanisms of food allergies, intolerances, and poisoning from dairy products, alcoholic beverages, and plant-based foods. Additionally, it delves into the toxic and allergic effects of heavy metals and medications, highlighting their impact on immune responses and systemic health.

One of the key strengths of this book is its integrative approach, combining in silico analyses, molecular studies, epidemiological data, and clinical perspectives. This multidisciplinary synthesis provides a robust framework for understanding how allergic and toxic reactions develop, their potential cross-reactivities, and the latest advancements in diagnostic and therapeutic modalities.

We believe that this book will serve as an invaluable resource for researchers, clinicians, and students in immunology, allergy, toxicology, and related disciplines. By fostering a deeper understanding of the intricate interactions between allergens, toxins, and the immune system, we hope to contribute to the development of more effective strategies for managing and preventing these conditions.

We extend our gratitude to the contributing authors for their expertise and dedication, as well as to our colleagues and institutions for their support in making this work possible. We hope this book will inspire further research and innovation in the fields of allergy, immunotoxicology, and clinical medicine.

Cartagena, Colombia — Marlon Gustavo Múnera Gómez
Monteria, Colombia — Juana Bustillo Arias
Bogotá, Colombia — Oscar Correa Jimenez
2025

Acknowledgment

I thank the Rafael Núñez University Corporation for supporting me in the development of this project.

Contents

About the Editors

Marlon Gustavo Múnera Gómez Biol, MSc, PhD, is a Professor in the Faculty of Health at Corporación Universitaria Rafael Nuñez in Cartagena, Colombia. He is also co-director of team research GINMUED, focused on the study of allergic and autoimmune responses. He was trained in murine models by ICGEB (The International Centre for Genetic Engineering and Biotechnology, Italy). He completed his immunological training and PhD at University of Cartagena. He sits on the editorial board as a guest for the *Journal of Frontiers in Allergy* and for the journal of *International Medical Research* and has published 52 papers, including 50 in international peer-reviewed journals and several book chapters related to biomedical sciences. He is a frequent invited keynote speaker at academic conferences and educational events across Colombia. He has supported vaccine design for immunotherapy to allergic diseases, at Institute for Immunological Research (Cartagena, Colombia).

Oscar Correa Jimenez is a highly experienced clinical immunologist with over a decade of practice in both adult and pediatric immunological and allergic conditions. He holds an MSc in Immunology and has specialized in treating complex immunological disorders. Dr. Correa-Jimenez has extensive expertise in clinical and translational research, particularly in immunology, molecular biology, and microbiology. Recognized as a national Key Opinion Leader (KOL) in Allergy and Clinical Immunology, he actively participates in international congresses and multinational research efforts on orphan diseases.

He has held prominent positions at various esteemed institutions, including the Unidad de Inmunología y Alergia del Mediterráneo-UDIAM IPS and the Fundación Neumológica Colombiana in Bogota, Colombia. His clinical work is complemented by his role as a consultant in clinical research and bioethics at the Universidad El Bosque. He has also served as a Medical Scientific Liaison at Takeda, enhancing his strategic and analytical skills in the pharmaceutical industry.

His academic contributions include teaching rotations in Allergy and Immunology for residents in Pediatrics, Pulmonology, and related fields at several universities. He has been an adjunct professor at the Universidad Nacional de Colombia, where he also co-led significant research groups.

He has authored numerous peer-reviewed publications and book chapters on immunological disorders, including topics like NLRP3-Associated Autoinflammation and autoimmune lymphoproliferative syndromes. His recent works have been published in prestigious journals such as the *Journal of Clinical Immunology* and *Cureus*.

Juana Bustillo Arias is an esteemed academic and researcher specializing in immunology and molecular biology. With a robust background in clinical and translational research, she has significantly contributed to understanding immune responses and their implications for human health. She holds a Master of Science degree in Immunology from Universidad De Cartagena, where her thesis focused on the association of chemokine and chemokine receptor expression with prostate cancer metastasis. She also completed her medical education at the same institution, receiving recognition as the best medical internship student. Her professional journey includes serving as a Clinical Immunologist at several prestigious institutions in Colombia, where she has led research groups in pulmonology, immunology in pediatrics, and genetics and molecular biology. Her work at Universidad Nacional de Colombia and Universidad de Cartagena has been pivotal in advancing research in these areas. Her research interests are reflected in her numerous peer-reviewed publications and book chapters, co-authoring significant works on topics such as NLRP3-associated autoinflammation, autoimmune lymphoproliferative syndromes, and respiratory comorbidities in patients with common variable immunodeficiency. Recognized for her contributions to the academic and research community, sh has presented her research at various international conferences and participated in multinational research collaborations, establishing herself as a key opinion leader in her field. For a complete list of her publications, please visit her profiles on Clarivate, Scopus, and Google Scholar.

Chapter 1
Intoxication and Allergenicity of *Cannabis sativa*

A. Sánchez, J. Sánchez, and Y. Emiliani

Introduction

Cannabis sativa is an annual herbaceous plant from the Cannabaceae family, belonging to the Rosales order, widely distributed around the world. It is easily recognized by its long, toothed, compound leaves. *C. sativa* is considered the most widely used drug globally, with 3.9% of the world's population (192 million people) consuming it for recreational and/or medical purposes [1]. Following the COVID-19 pandemic, isolation contributed to an increase in its use to cope with negative events [2, 3].

The preparations of *C. sativa* vary according to its use, including dry components, paste, liquids, oil, or resin, which can be ingested, vaporized, applied as ointments, in capsules, or smoked [4]. These preparations can use the whole plant or specific parts such as leaves, flowers, or stems. Although promoted as a "harmless"

A. Sánchez (✉)
Group of Clinical and Experimental Allergy (GACE), University of Antioquia, Medellín, Colombia

Group of Medicine Investigation (GINUMED), Corporation University Rafael Núñez, Faculty of Exact and Natural Sciences, Cartagena, Colombia

Pharmaceutical, Cosmetic and Food Technology Research Group (GIFTCA). University of Cartagena, Cartagena, Colombia
e-mail: Andres.sanchez@curnvirtual.edu.co

J. Sánchez
Group of Clinical and Experimental Allergy (GACE), University of Antioquia, Medellín, Colombia

Y. Emiliani
Group of Medicine Investigation (GINUMED), Corporation University Rafael Núñez, Faculty of Exact and Natural Sciences, Cartagena, Colombia

M. G. Múnera Gómez et al. (eds.), *Allergies, Poisoning and Intolerance to Common Substances*, https://doi.org/10.1007/978-3-031-93658-6_1

natural plant, its consumption has been associated with intoxication, contamination, and allergies.

C. sativa contains more than 400 components, 60 of which are cannabinoids with psychoactive effects on the central nervous system and the immune system. The most studied components are 9-tetrahydrocannabinol (THC) and cannabidiol (CBD), both associated with marijuana intoxication. This intoxication can be chronic due to prolonged use or acute due to excessive THC consumption. Symptoms include irritability, disorientation, hallucinations, depersonalization, and psychosis, as well as digestive, cardiac, respiratory, endocrine, and immunological effects.

Allergy to *Cannabis* has gained relevance in health, although its prevalence is underestimated due to illegality in many countries and the lack of reliable diagnostic methods [3, 5, 6]. Allergic manifestations include atopic rhinoconjunctivitis, allergic keratoconjunctivitis, hypersensitivity pneumonitis, asthma exacerbations, skin reactions, pruritus, dermatitis, angioedema, contact urticaria, respiratory symptoms, and anaphylaxis [6, 8–11].

With the legalization of *Cannabis* for recreational and/or pharmacological use in several countries, an increase in intoxications and hypersensitivities to *C. sativa* is expected. The similarity of symptoms complicates proper clinical differentiation and management. This chapter focuses on describing *C. sativa* intoxications and allergies, the triggering components, and the necessary diagnostic tests for their differentiation.

Cannabis sativa Intoxication

The psychoactive effects, low cost, and easy acquisition of *Cannabis sativa* make it one of the most widely consumed drugs worldwide. Additionally, changes in legalization in countries like Canada and several states in the United States have led to an increase in marijuana use, even among pediatric and juvenile populations, which previously had very low usage rates. The availability and variety of its forms have made its consumption more attractive.

Various studies have evaluated the acute and chronic harmful effects of marijuana consumption and its components, identifying two main ones: 9-tetrahydrocannabinol (THC) and cannabidiol (CBD).

9-Tetrahydrocannabinol (THC)

THC is the primary psychoactive constituent of marijuana, first described as a psychoactive molecule by Gaoni & Mechoulam in 1964 [12]. This liposoluble cannabinoid is highly protein-bound and has a distribution volume of 2.5–3.5 L/kg. It is considered the principal psychoactive molecule of *C. sativa* due to its ability to bind to brain cannabinoid receptors (CB-1 and CB-2), transient receptor potential ion channels (TRP), and peroxisome proliferator-activated receptors gamma (PPARγ), inducing sedative, hallucinogenic, and stimulant effects. These effects depend on the administration method, dose, and exposure time. Adverse symptoms can also occur in the nervous, ophthalmological, gastrointestinal, and cardiovascular systems.

Pharmacokinetics vary by administration route (oral, inhaled, rectal, or vaginal). Inhalation shows a route similar to intravenous administration. For THC, psychoactive effects coincide with serum detection, which can occur within 15–30 min and last up to 4 h. Due to its liposoluble characteristics, THC is rapidly metabolized. Ingestion peaks occur between 1 and 2 h, with psychoactive effects starting between 30 min and 3 h and lasting up to 12 h, depending on the amount consumed. Bioavailability ranges from 10% to 35% depending on inhalation strength, which is significantly higher than ingestion (5–20%) due to gastric acid degradation and subsequent liver metabolism. Minimum THC concentrations required for psychoactive effects range from 2 to 3 mg when inhaled and 5 to 20 mg when ingested, but these concentrations tend to increase with prolonged use [12, 13].

THC metabolism primarily occurs in the liver via the cytochrome P450 pathway, involving CYP2C9, CYP2C19, and CYP3A4. THC is converted into its primary active metabolite 11-hydroxy-THC (11-OH-THC) and the inactive metabolite 11-carboxy-THC (11-COOH-THC). The half-life of THC varies from 25 to 36 h, and its metabolites are excreted in feces (65%) and urine (20%) [14, 15]. Additionally, THC can cross the placenta and be found in breast milk, potentially causing brain toxicity in infants [16].

Cannabidiol (CBD)

Cannabidiol (CBD), or 2-[(6R)-6-isopropenyl-3-methyl-2-cyclohexen-1-yl]-5-pentyl-1,3-benzenediol, was identified in 1940 by Adams et al., with its structure described in 1963 (REF). Similar to THC, this molecule acts on central nervous system cannabinoid receptors CB-1 and CB-2, transient receptor potential cation channels (TRPV1), peroxisome proliferator-activated receptors (PPARγ), and serotonin 1 receptors (5-HT1A). However, it is not considered a psychoactive molecule. CBD functions as a CB-1 antagonist and a CB-2 inverse agonist and activates PPARγ, which explains its anti-inflammatory properties [17]. Like THC, CBD is metabolized in the liver via cytochrome P450 enzymes, specifically CYP2C19, and the UDP-glucuronosyltransferase isoforms UGT1A7, UGT1A9, and UGT2B7.

Intoxication occurs from excessive or constant consumption of marijuana and its cannabinoids, often accompanied by the inclusion of other substances, such as cocaine. The manifestations of toxicity depend on the amount and duration of consumption. Infants, who typically access these drugs through a family member, can present a range of symptoms from irritability and altered mental state to encephalopathy and coma. Lavi et al. [17] studied three cases of infants aged 8–14 months who had accidental intoxication, describing lethargy, irritability, vomiting, and unconsciousness. The authors emphasize the need to train healthcare professionals on cannabis intoxication and suggest conducting appropriate clinical tests if sensory diminution is observed. The risk of consuming marijuana orally lies in its delayed effect, leading consumers to ingest more doses, affecting various systems.

Allergy to *Cannabis sativa*

Cannabis sativa allergens can trigger type I and type IV hypersensitivity reactions. To date, the WHO/IUIS Allergen Nomenclature Subcommittee has accepted four allergens [18], distributed in various parts of the plant, such as pollen, seeds, and leaves. The nonspecific lipid transfer protein (nsLTP), Can s 3, is considered the main allergen in Europe [19]. Other allergens identified with IgE binding capability and potential to trigger allergic responses include the oxygen-evolving enhancer protein (Can s 4), cannabis profilin (Can s 2), and Bet v 1 homolog (Can s 5) [20, 21]. Other components of cannabis, such as delta-9-tetrahydrocannabinol, thaumatin-like protein, and ribulose-1,5-bisphosphate carboxylase/oxygenase (Can s RuBisCO), are being studied as potential allergens [22, 23].

The first reported hypersensitivity reaction to cannabis was described in 1971, involving a woman who developed an anaphylactic reaction after smoking a cannabis-containing cigarette. Since then, many reports have been published on this topic [24]. However, little is known about specific cannabis allergens. Currently, only four proteins have been officially recognized as allergens by the International Union of Immunological Societies (IUIS): the nonspecific lipid transfer protein (nsLTP, Can s 3), profilin (Can s 2), oxygen-evolving enhancer protein 2 (Can s 4), and pathogenesis-related protein 10 homolog (PR10, Can s 5) [20, 21]. Other potential allergens, such as thaumatin-like protein (TLP) and ribulose-1,5-bisphosphate carboxylase/oxygenase (RuBisCO), are also considered relevant in the sensitization to *Cannabis sativa*.

Cannabis allergens can cause cross-reactions, primarily with vegetables. However, knowledge about cross-reactions with plant-derived foods and their association with cannabis allergy is limited. As far as we know, this is the first in silico study exploring the possible cross-reactivity between plant sources and potential cannabis allergens through molecular mimicry.

Cross-reactivity between cannabis allergens and other plant sources has been confirmed. For example, sensitization to *C. sativa* extract has been observed in patients allergic to white birch pollen, tomatoes, latex, tobacco, and some alcoholic beverages, indicating that it can induce symptoms in these patients and may act as a primary sensitizing allergen [23, 25, 26].

The first reports of allergenicity related to cannabis allergens describe cases of plant-derived food allergies. Gamboa et al. reported a case of a 28-year-old man who, following a cannabis allergy, experienced anaphylaxis after consuming pepper, fig, and tomato. Additionally, the patient developed contact urticaria from peach skin and oral allergy syndrome from almonds, eggplant, and chestnut [19]. Other studies have also reported an association with tomato allergy and suggested a link with tobacco allergy [7, 25]. Subsequently, cannabis allergy has been associated with symptoms after ingesting hazelnuts, walnuts, peanuts, corn, nectarines, cherries, kiwi, avocado, apples, as well as wine, beer, and latex exposure.

The nonspecific lipid transfer protein (nsLTP, Can s 3) is considered the main allergen of *C. sativa* in Europe and the major cannabis allergen related to plant-derived food allergies [19, 27, 28]. Diagnostic tests based on Can s 3 account for 80% and 60% of positive and negative values of *C. sativa* in Europe [28]. LTPs are widespread in the plant kingdom and present in many vegetables and fruits. Thus, multiple food allergens belong to the same protein family, such as Pru p 3 (peach), Mal d 3 (apple), and Mor n 3 (mulberry), considered pan-allergens. Due to their similar chemical structure, cross-reactivity is common among them [29]. However, a few studies have evaluated the cross-reactive potential of Can s 3. nsLTPs are highly stable food allergens associated with both raw and cooked plant foods. Cross-reactivity between rCan s 3 and Pru p 3 was confirmed through IgE inhibition experiments in a group of European patients, where 31.3% of the serum with sIgE for rCan s 3 also had positive sIgE values for Pru p 3 [27]. The exposure route to cannabis allergens like Can s 3 is variable, and thus, possible cross-reactivity is not exclusive to food allergens; it can also occur with ornamental, medicinal, and forage plants, such as Hevea latex.

Faber et al. [30] analyzed the role of Hev b 12 in five patients with natural rubber latex (NRL) allergy. They demonstrated that patients sensitized to Hev b 12 with a positive basophil activation test showed sIgE reactivity to rPru p 3, and only one patient showed positive sIgE to Can s 3 without reactivity to other latex allergens. They suggest that Hev b 12 is unlikely to be the primary sensitizer, but other sources such as cannabis or peach could be the triggers of allergic symptoms.

Can s 2 belongs to the profilin family, and its allergenicity was described by Ebo et al., who studied the IgE binding capacity to cannabis profilin in five patients from Belgium and Germany using an IgE-binding assay with a cytometric bead array [21]. Cross-reactivity among members of the profilin family has been well studied [21, 31–33]. These proteins are actin-binding and ubiquitous in plants, found in pollen, fruits, vegetables, and forage plants such as *Hevea* latex.

In the same study by Ebo et al., the allergenicity of Can s 5 was examined, demonstrating an sIgE binding capacity to the Bet v 1 homolog [21]. Bet v 1 homologs belong to pathogenesis-related proteins (PR-10) and show significant cross-reactivity with pollen from fruits and vegetables. Sensitization to the cannabis allergen Bet v 1 homolog Can s 5 occurs in individuals with cannabis allergy, but it is unclear if these patients also have pollen-food syndrome (PFS) or oral allergy syndrome (OAS) [3]. Our study found that 16 Bet v 1 homologs with identity to Can s 5 belonged to fruit plants in the Rosaceae family (mainly the genera Prunus, Pyrus, and Malus domestica), which have shown cross-reactivity with other edible fruits [34–36].

The diversity of species and the similarity among profilin and Bet v 1 homologs present a challenge in understanding their relevance in cross-sensitization. Therefore, in vivo and in vitro studies are necessary to confirm their role in the development of oral allergy syndrome and their potential contribution to cross-reactivity of Bet v 1 homologs.

Similarly, the oxygen-evolving enhancer protein Can s 4, the thaumatin-like protein, and RuBiCo showed significant homology with a diverse range of plants in our study, suggesting potential new allergenic sources. Therefore, further studies are necessary to corroborate their relevance as *C. sativa* allergens in both cross-reactive food allergies and contact reactions.

In silico analyses are recognized as the initial step in research, allowing for prioritization of resources and facilitating a preliminary approach to expected outcomes. These studies form the basis for more robust projects, such as using biological models. Describing potential epitopes of *Cannabis sativa* allergens opens the door to exploring IgE binding sites and considering specific mutagenicity studies as opportunities for immunotherapy treatments. Confirmation through in vitro studies could also lead to a better understanding of the pathophysiology of allergies to various plant sources, such as oral allergy syndrome.

Differential Diagnosis Between Intoxication and Allergy to *C. sativa*

The conventional drug test in urine samples is used to detect metabolites of tetrahydrocannabinol (THC), especially THC carboxylase, with lower limits of quantification ranging from 20 to 100 ng/mL. Although the likelihood of obtaining positive results in adolescents and adults is high, exhaustive research in the pediatric context is lacking. Various agents can generate false positives for THC, such as dronabinol, efavirenz, proton pump inhibitors (PPIs), hemp seed oil, nonsteroidal anti-inflammatory drugs (NSAIDs), and baby care products [37].

The incidence of false positive results decreases significantly in analytical laboratories with gas chromatography capabilities. Additionally, positive results for THC carboxylase can persist up to 10 days after weekly use and up to 30 days after intensive daily use. This variability in exposure chronology complicates the correlation between the timing of the test and the severity of THC intoxication [37, 38].

On the other hand, the foremost method for diagnosing cannabis allergy lies in collecting the patient's clinical history. Unfortunately, once anamnesis is established, standardized allergy tests are not always feasible due to the scarcity of commercially available extracts. Consequently, skin prick tests (SPT) using cannabis plant components often emerge as the only viable alternative when accessible. The complexity of the situation intensifies because, despite the essential nature of these tests for diagnosis, acquiring cannabis plant materials is challenging in many countries, hindering the tests and achieving an accurate diagnosis [39, 40].

Additionally, component-resolved diagnosis can enhance accuracy, particularly using Can s 3, which accounts for 70% of sensitization in European regions. Unfortunately, the predictive capacity in regions like Latin America or North America is unknown, so other *C. sativa* allergens might play a significant role in IgE binding [39].

Cell-based tests such as ex vivo basophil activation tests (BAT) and mast cell activation tests (pMAT) can also be useful. Unlike traditional sIgE binding assays, they reflect the in vivo situation and, along with SPT, can help detect sensitization to compounds with carbohydrate determinants and enable safe evaluation of recombinants. Thus, a negative SPT or BAT has good predictive value, but a positive result in one of these tests warrants complementary diagnostics [40].

Conclusion

In conclusion, we identified a high identity between *Cannabis sativa* allergens and various food and contact proteins, most of which are major allergen sources. We also described potential antigenic sites among cannabis allergens, where the high identity between these proteins from different species and cannabis allergens suggests possible cross-reactivity due to molecular mimicry. These findings underscore the need for in vitro and in vivo studies to confirm the allergenic potential of cannabis allergens.

Glossary

Glossary of Acronyms

BAT (Basophil Activation Test) A test that measures basophil activation to diagnose allergies.

CBD (Cannabidiol) A non-psychoactive cannabinoid known for its anti-inflammatory properties.

CB1 (Cannabinoid Receptor 1) A receptor in the central nervous system that binds cannabinoids, primarily THC.

CB2 (Cannabinoid Receptor 2) A receptor in the immune system that binds cannabinoids, involved in anti-inflammatory responses.

GINUMED (Group of Medicine Investigation) A research group at Corporation University Rafael Núñez, Cartagena, Colombia.

GIFTCA (Pharmaceutical Cosmetic and Food Technology Research Group) A research group at the University of Cartagena, Colombia.

IUIS (International Union of Immunological Societies) An organization that recognizes and names allergens.

LTP (Lipid Transfer Protein) A major allergen found in various plants, including Cannabis sativa.

OEEP2 (Oxygen-Evolving Enhancer Protein 2) A protein allergen found in Cannabis sativa.

PPARγ (Peroxisome Proliferator-Activated Receptor Gamma) A receptor that cannabinoids can activate, contributing to their anti-inflammatory effects.

PR10 (Pathogenesis-Related Protein 10) A protein family that includes allergenic proteins in Cannabis sativa.

pMAT (Mast Cell Activation Test) A test used to identify mast cell activation in response to allergens.

Pru p 3 A lipid transfer protein from peach, known to cross-react with cannabis allergens.

rCan s 3 Recombinant Can s 3, a nonspecific lipid transfer protein allergen from Cannabis sativa.

RuBisCO (Ribulose-1,5-bisphosphate carboxylase/oxygenase) An enzyme that can act as an allergen in Cannabis sativa.

SPT (Skin Prick Test) A diagnostic method for identifying allergies by exposing the skin to potential allergens.

THC (Tetrahydrocannabinol) The primary psychoactive component of cannabis, responsible for its intoxicating effects.

TRPV1 (Transient Receptor Potential Vanilloid 1) A receptor involved in the detection and regulation of body temperature and pain, activated by cannabinoids.

UGT (UDP-Glucuronosyltransferase) A family of enzymes involved in the metabolism of cannabinoids like CBD in the liver.

WHO (World Health Organization) An international public health agency involved in the nomenclature and classification of allergens.

Glossary of Terms

Allergens Substances in cannabis that can trigger allergic reactions, such as Can s 3, Can s 2, Can s 4, and Can s 5.

Anaphylaxis A severe, potentially life-threatening allergic reaction.

Atopic Rhinoconjunctivitis An allergic condition affecting the nose and eyes, commonly triggered by cannabis.

Basophil Activation Test (BAT) A test that measures basophil activation to diagnose allergies.

Bioavailability The degree and rate at which a substance, like THC, is absorbed into the bloodstream.

Cannabinoids Chemical compounds found in cannabis, affecting the central nervous and immune systems. Over 60 cannabinoids are identified, including THC and CBD.

Cannabis Sativa An herbaceous plant from the Cannabaceae family, widely used for recreational and medical purposes.

Cross-reactivity The phenomenon where cannabis allergens react with proteins from other plant sources, causing allergies.

CBD (Cannabidiol) A non-psychoactive cannabinoid known for its anti-inflammatory properties.

Cytochrome P450 A family of enzymes involved in the metabolism of THC and CBD in the liver.

Hypersensitivity An exaggerated immune response to cannabis, leading to allergic reactions.

Intoxication The state of being affected by the psychoactive components of cannabis, causing symptoms like irritability, hallucinations, and psychosis.

Legalization The process of making the use of cannabis legal, which can impact rates of consumption and related health issues.

Mast Cell Activation Test (pMAT) A test used to identify mast cell activation in response to allergens.

Metabolism The process by which the body breaks down substances, such as the liver's role in metabolizing cannabinoids.

nsLTP (Nonspecific Lipid Transfer Protein) A major allergen in cannabis associated with food allergies.

Pollen-Food Syndrome An allergic reaction to pollen and certain foods, often linked to cannabis allergens.

Psychoactive Effects Mental and behavioral changes caused by substances like THC, including euphoria and hallucinations.

Skin Prick Test (SPT) A diagnostic method for identifying allergies by exposing the skin to potential allergens.

THC (Tetrahydrocannabinol) The primary psychoactive component of cannabis, responsible for its intoxicating effects.

References

1. Lozano I. The therapeutic use of Cannabis sativa (L.) in Arabic medicine. J Cannabis Ther. 2001;1(1):63–70.
2. Bartel SJ, Sherry SB, Stewart SH. Self-isolation: a significant contributor to cannabis use during the COVID-19 pandemic. Subst Abus. 2020;41(4):409–12.
3. Skypala IJ, Jeimy S, Brucker H, Nayak AP, Decuyper II, Bernstein JA, et al. Cannabis-related allergies: an international overview and consensus recommendations. Allergy [Internet]. 2022;77(7):2038–52. Available from: https://onlinelibrary.wiley.com/doi/10.1111/all.15237
4. Chandra S, Lata H, ElSohly MA. Cannabis sativa L.—botany and biotechnology. Cannabis sativa L—botany and. Biotechnology. 2017:1–474.
5. Jackson B, Cleto E, Jeimy S, Jeimy S. An emerging allergen: Cannabis sativa allergy in a climate of recent legalization. Allergy Asthma Clin Immunol [Internet]. 2020;16(1):1–6. https://doi.org/10.1186/s13223-020-00447-9.
6. Chatkin JM, Zani-Silva L, Ferreira I, Zamel N. Cannabis-Associated Asthma and Allergies. Vol. 56, Clinical Reviews in Allergy and Immunology. Humana Press Inc; 2019. p. 196–206.
7. Armentia A, Castrodeza J, Ruiz-Muñoz P, Martínez-Quesada J, Postigo I, Herrero M, et al. Allergic hypersensitivity to cannabis in patients with allergy and illicit drug users. Allergol Immunopathol (Madr). 2011;39(5):271–9.
8. Chatkin JM, Zani-Silva L, Ferreira I, Zamel N. Cannabis-associated asthma and allergies. Clin Rev Allergy Immunol. 2019;56(2):196–206.
9. Decuyper II, Faber MA, Lapeere H, Mertens C, Rihs HP, van Gasse AL, et al. Cannabis allergy: a diagnostic challenge. Vol. 73, Allergy: European Journal of Allergy and Clinical Immunology. Blackwell Publishing Ltd; 2018. p. 1911–4.

10. Decuyper II, van Gasse AL, Cop N, Sabato V, Faber MA, Mertens C, et al. Cannabis sativa allergy: looking through the fog, vol. 72. Allergy: European Journal of Allergy and Clinical Immunology. Blackwell Publishing Ltd; 2017. p. 201–6.
11. Stepaniuk P, Kanani A. Selective cannabis strain allergy in a patient presenting with a local allergic reaction. Allergy Asthma Clin Immunol. 2021;17(1)
12. Wong KU, Baum CR. Acute cannabis toxicity, vol. 35. [Internet]; 2019. p. 799. www.pec--online.com
13. Noble MJ, Hedberg K, Hendrickson RG. Acute cannabis toxicity. Clin Toxicol. 2019;57(8):735–42.
14. Grotenhermen F. Pharmacokinetics and pharmacodynamics of cannabinoids. Clin Pharmacokinet. 2003;42:327–60.
15. Lucas CJ, Galettis P, Schneider J. The pharmacokinetics and the pharmacodynamics of cannabinoids. Vol. 84, British Journal of Clinical Pharmacology. Blackwell Publishing Ltd; 2018. p. 2477–82.
16. Wymore EM, Palmer C, Wang GS, Metz TD, Bourne DWA, Sempio C, et al. Persistence of Δ-9-tetrahydrocannabinol in human breast Milk. JAMA Pediatr. 2021;175(6):632–4.
17. Lavi E, Rekhtman D, Berkun Y, Wexler I. Sudden onset unexplained encephalopathy in infants: think of cannabis intoxication. Eur J Pediatr. 2016;175(3):417–20.
18. Sudharson S, Kalic T, Hafner C, Breiteneder H. Newly defined allergens in the WHO/IUIS allergen nomenclature database during 01/2019-03/2021, vol. 76. Allergy: European Journal of Allergy and Clinical Immunology. John Wiley and Sons Inc; 2021. p. 3359–73.
19. Gamboa P, Sanchez-Monge R, Sanz ML, Palacín A, Salcedo G, Diaz-Perales A. Sensitization to Cannabis sativa caused by a novel allergenic lipid transfer protein, can s 3. J Allergy Clin Immunol. 2007;120(6):1459–60.
20. Decuyper II, Rihs HP, Mertens CH, van Gasse AL, Elst J, de Puysseleyr L, et al. A new cannabis allergen in northwestern Europe: the oxygen-evolving enhancer protein 2 (OEEP2). J Allergy Clin Immunol In Pract. 2020;8(7):2421–2424.e2.
21. Ebo DG, Decuyper II, Rihs HP, Mertens C, van Gasse AL, van der Poorten MLM, et al. IgE-binding and mast cell–activating capacity of the homologue of the major birch pollen allergen and profilin from Cannabis sativa. Journal of Allergy and Clinical Immunology: In Practice [Internet]. 2021;9(6):2509–2512.e3. https://doi.org/10.1016/j.jaip.2021.02.012.
22. Larramendi CH, López-Matas MÁ, Ferrer Á, Huertas ÁJ, Pagán JA, Navarro LÁ, et al. Prevalence of sensitization to cannabis sativa. Lipid-transfer and thaumatin-like proteins are relevant allergens. Int Arch Allergy Immunol. 2013;162(2):115–22.
23. Nayak AP, Green BJ, Sussman G, Berlin N, Lata H, Chandra S, et al. Characterization of Cannabis sativa allergens. Ann Allergy Asthma Immunol [Internet]. 2013;111(1):32–37.e4. https://doi.org/10.1016/j.anai.2013.04.018.
24. Liskow B, Liss JL, Parker CW, Louis S. Allergy to marihuana [Internet]. Ann Intern Med. 1971. Available from: http://annals.org/pdfaccess.ashx?url=/data/journals/aim/19454/;75:571.
25. de Larramendi CH, Carnés J, García-Abujeta JL, García-Endrino A, Muñoz-Palomino E, Huertas ÁJ, et al. Sensitization and allergy to Cannabis sativa leaves in a population of tomato (Lycopersicon esculentum)-sensitized patients. Int Arch Allergy Immunol. 2008;146(3):195–202.
26. Drouet M, Hoppe A, Moreau AS, Bonneau JC, Leclere JM, le Sellin J. Cannabis and crossed allergy with food. Revue de Pneumologie Clinique Elsevier Masson SAS. 2017;73:290–3.
27. Rihs HP, Armentia A, Sander I, Brüning T, Raulf M, Varga R. IgE-binding properties of a recombinant lipid transfer protein from Cannabis sativa. Ann Allergy Asthma Immunolgy [Internet]. 2014;113(2):233–4. https://doi.org/10.1016/j.anai.2014.05.022.
28. Decuyper II, van Gasse AL, Faber MA, Elst J, Mertens C, Rihs HP, et al. Exploring the diagnosis and profile of cannabis allergy. J Allergy Clin Immunol: In Practice [Internet]. 2019;7(3):983–989.e5. https://doi.org/10.1016/j.jaip.2018.09.017.
29. Skypala IJ, Asero R, Barber D, Cecchi L, Diaz Perales A, Hoffmann-Sommergruber K, et al. Non-specific lipid-transfer proteins: allergen structure and function, cross-reactivity,

sensitization, and epidemiology, vol. 11. Clinical and Translational Allergy. John Wiley and Sons Inc; 2021.
30. Faber MA, Sabato V, Bridts CH, Nayak A, Beezhold DH, Ebo DG. Clinical relevance of the Hevea brasiliensis lipid transfer protein Hev b 12. J Allergy Clin Immunol. 2015;135(6):1645–8.
31. Foong RX, Dantzer JA, Wood RA, Santos AF. Improving diagnostic accuracy in food allergy. J Allergy Clin Immunol In Pract. 2021;9(1):71–80.
32. Yagami A, Ebisawa M. New findings, pathophysiology, and antigen analysis in pollen-food allergy syndrome. Curr Opin Allergy Clin Immunol. 2019;19(3):218–23.
33. Rosace D, Gomez-Casado C, Fernandez P, Perez-Gordo M, del Carmen DM, Vega A, et al. Profilin-mediated food-induced allergic reactions are associated with oral epithelial remodeling. J Allergy Clin Immunol. 2019;143(2):681–90.
34. Gamboa PM, Cáceres O, Antepara I, Sánchez-Monge R, Ahrazem O, Salcedo G, et al. Two different profiles of peach allergy in the north of Spain. Allergy: European. J Allergy Clin Immunol. 2007;62(4):408–14.
35. Wiche R, Gubesch M, Onig HK, Otisch KF, Hoffmann A, Wangorsch A, et al. Molecular basis of pollen-related food allergy: identification of a second cross-reactive IgE epitope on Pru av 1, the major cherry (Prunus avium) allergen. Biochem J. 2005;385:319.
36. Karamloo F, Scheurer S, Wangorsch A, May S, Haustein D, Vieths S. Pyr c 1, the major allergen from pear (Pyrus communis), is a new member of the Bet v 1 allergen family. J Chromatogr B Biomed Sci Appl. 2001;756(1–2):281–93.
37. Turner AR, Spurling BC, Agrawal S. Marijuana toxicity. In: StatPearls [internet]. StatPearls Publishing; 2023.
38. Alghamdi AM, Samman OY, Bahader WK, Bakhsh TA, Altuwaylib SM, Haider MA, et al. Cannabinoid acute intoxication, diagnosis, and management. Int J Pharm Res Allied Sci. 2021;10(4):42.
39. Toscano A, Elst J, van der Poorten ML, Beyens M, Heremans K, Decuyper II, et al. Establishing diagnostic strategies for cannabis allergy. Expert Rev Clin Immunol. 2022;18(10):1015–22.
40. Decuyper II, Van Gasse AL, Faber MA, Elst J, Mertens C, Rihs HP, et al. Exploring the diagnosis and profile of cannabis allergy. J Allergy Clin Immunol Pract. 2019;7(3):983–9.

Chapter 2
Anisakis Simplex: Parasitism and Allergy

Velky Ahumada and Juan Ricardo Urrego

Introduction

The larvae of the nematode family Anisakidae can infect a wide range of commercially significant fish species. However, their public health relevance lies in the fact that humans can become accidental hosts when consuming fish contaminated with these parasites. In humans, the infection usually manifests as a series of gastrointestinal symptoms [1]. However, in some cases, these symptoms are not confined to the gastrointestinal tract, as the larvae can penetrate the digestive wall and reach organs such as the liver, pancreas, ovaries, and lymph nodes. In these locations, the larvae can remain latent until they are gradually degraded [2].

Among the Anisakidae family, several species are of interest, with *Anisakis simplex* being the most studied. This species is a source of potent allergens, and in susceptible individuals, consuming fish contaminated with this parasite can trigger allergic reactions [3, 4]. The first report of allergy caused by *A. simplex* was published in Japan in the 1990s. Since then, numerous studies worldwide have examined the allergy to this nematode, considering it a risk factor for developing food allergies, especially in cultures like Peruvian or Japanese, where raw fish consumption is common [5, 6]. However, with the globalization of cuisine and the fishing

V. Ahumada (✉) J. R. Urrego
Research Group on Pharmaceutical, Cosmetic and Food Technology, Faculty of Exact and Natural Sciences, Universidad de Cartagena, Cartagena, Colombia

Research Group on Pharmaceutical, Cosmetic and Food Technology, Universidad de Cartagena, Cartagena, Bolívar, Colombia
e-mail: vahumadac@unicartagena.edu.co; jurregoa1@unicartagena.edu.co

M. G. Múnera Gómez et al. (eds.), *Allergies, Poisoning and Intolerance to Common Substances*, https://doi.org/10.1007/978-3-031-93658-6_2

industry, the risk of human infection by anisakiasis seems underestimated in developed countries [7].

To date, 14 allergens of *Anisakis simplex* have been officially reported by the Allergen Nomenclature Subcommittee of the World Health Organization and the International Union of Immunological Societies (WHO/IUIS). This chapter will discuss *Anisakis simplex*, the clinical manifestations of anisakiasis, its life cycle, the allergic reactions it induces, and its allergens.

Life Cycle of *Anisakis simplex*

Anisakis simplex is a helminth, classified as a roundworm with a non-segmented body, belonging to the class Nematoda. This nematode is whitish, almost transparent, and small, reaching a length of approximately three centimeters. It belongs to the family Anisakidae, which includes 24 species of the genus *Anisakis* [7], among which *Anisakis simplex* is the primary cause of foodborne infections and allergic reactions [8].

Anisakis simplex is an intestinal parasite of marine mammals, fish, and some birds. Its biological cycle occurs in an aquatic environment and requires one or more intermediate hosts (see Fig. 2.1). This cycle includes an adult form and four

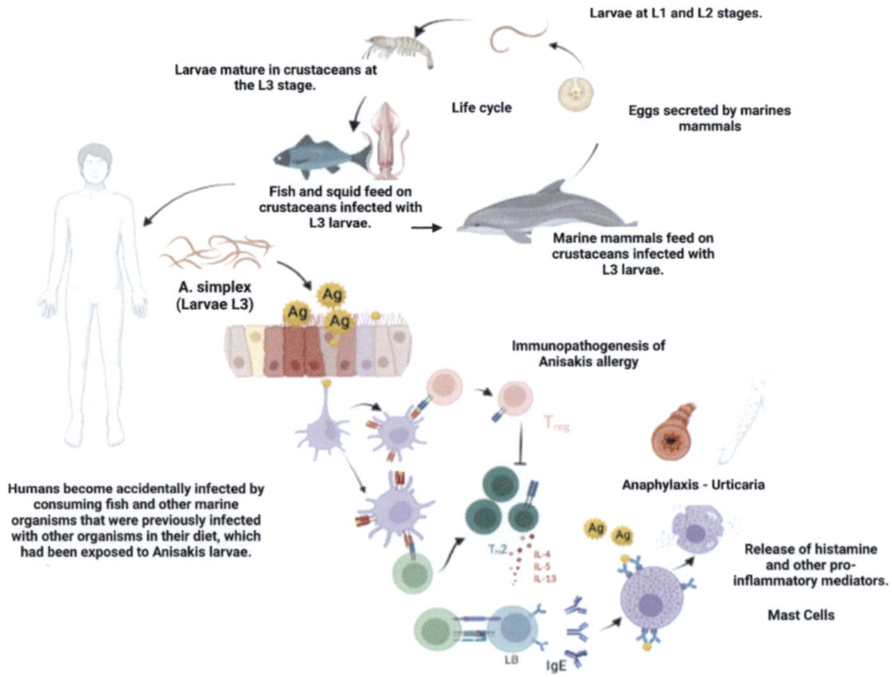

Fig. 2.1 Life cycle of *Anisakis simplex* and immunopathogenesis of *A. simplex* allergy

larval stages. The first larval stage (L1) consists of eggs that come from the feces of definitive hosts (fish, marine mammals, and some birds), where the parasite develops into its adult form. Free in the sea, the eggs hatch into the second larval stage (L2), which can be ingested by small planktonic crustaceans, constituting the first intermediate host. These crustaceans are then eaten by other fish and cephalopods, becoming the second intermediate hosts, in which the third larval stage (L3) develops. This larva can pass from one fish or cephalopod to another and, when ingested by larger marine mammals or fish, it reaches its adult stage, releasing eggs into the environment through the feces of the definitive host, thus closing the biological cycle [7].

Humans become accidental hosts when they ingest the L3 larva. In humans, these parasites cannot reach the adult stage, remaining as they were ingested in the third larval stage. Many marine species act as secondary hosts capable of transmitting L3 larvae to humans. These include species such as hake, mackerel, cod, sardine, anchovy, herring, and salmon [9]. In these fish, the parasites can be found free in the intestine, penetrating the intestinal wall, or encapsulated in various organs or muscles [10]. In the L3 stage, the *Anisakis simplex* larva reaches 2–3 cm in length and is usually found in the digestive tract when the fish is alive [7].

Clinical Manifestations of Anisakiasis

Anisakiasis is an infection caused by the helminth *Anisakis simplex*. This parasite can infect humans, particularly those who consume raw or undercooked fish containing L3 stage larvae [11]. The main symptoms of the infection include epigastric pain accompanied by nausea and vomiting [1, 12]. In some individuals, sensitization to Anisakis antigens can trigger an allergic intestinal reaction, resulting in symptoms such as urticaria, angioedema, and anaphylaxis following the ingestion and/or exposure to infected fish [1, 12]. Additionally, individuals exposed to the parasite's proteins can become sensitized through contact or inhalation of the allergens. Susceptible individuals may develop IgE-mediated allergic reactions ranging from urticaria to anaphylactic shock [1, 13].

Digestive Conditions

When raw or insufficiently cooked fish contaminated with *Anisakis simplex* larvae is consumed, the larvae remain alive and are ingested along with the fish, reaching the stomach or intestines of the person. Upon reaching the digestive tract, several outcomes are possible. The first possibility is that the larva passes through the digestive tract without causing any issues, as these larvae are not adapted to the human body and are eliminated through defecation. However, the larvae can also attach to the walls of the digestive tract, perforating the superficial layer and causing an inflammatory process at the implantation sites. This manifests as abdominal pain, with or without vomiting and diarrhea. Symptoms typically appear between 24 and 48 h after consuming the fish [14].

The intestinal form of the infection often follows a chronic course, developing abscesses with remnants of Anisakis in the intestinal wall. This can lead to abdominal pain and changes in bowel habits, sometimes causing acute appendicitis or intestinal obstruction [15]. However, in most patients, anisakiasis is self-limiting, resolving spontaneously as the larva is expelled. In some cases, where intestinal complications arise, surgical intervention may be necessary [16].

Diagnosis of Anisakiasis

Radiography and ultrasound can be useful in diagnosing anisakiasis, but definitive diagnosis is achieved through endoscopic visualization of the larvae. This technique allows for the direct observation of larvae attached to the gastric mucosa and their extraction via the endoscope, often alleviating clinical symptoms. Rarely, parasites have been found in organs other than the digestive tract (liver, lung, spleen, pancreas) due to larval migration from the intestine to distant sites [17].

Serological diagnosis of *A. simplex* is challenging due to the high cross-reactivity of its proteins with those of other nematodes. Most of these antigens contain shared protein and carbohydrate epitopes, even with phylogenetically unrelated organisms like insects. Cross-reactivity is suspected to be responsible for the "false positives" of specific IgE detected in individuals without clinical histories of Anisakis allergy. An alternative to this problem is using deglycosylated specific allergens captured by monoclonal antibodies in techniques such as capture ELISA [18]. Another diagnostic option is the basophil activation test, which has shown high diagnostic accuracy (92.45%) and specificity (100%) against Anisakis allergy [19]. Recently, a study using purified *A. simplex* allergens found that specific IgE seropositivity to the Ani s 1 allergen could be a biomarker for detecting patients at risk of severe allergic reactions [20].

Allergic Reactions to *Anisakis simplex*

Anisakis simplex, a helminth of the nematode class, has been extensively studied in allergology due to its potent allergens [21]. Allergic reactions induced by this helminth are primarily characterized by acute generalized urticaria, with or without swelling (angioedema), and sometimes severe symptoms such as anaphylactic shock [22]. These symptoms typically appear between 4 and 72 h after consuming infected fish and may or may not be accompanied by gastrointestinal symptoms. Sensitized individuals react to the secreted or excreted products (allergens) of *Anisakis simplex* larvae, leading to an allergic response that can vary in intensity based on individual sensitivity and the number of antigens present [23].

There is a close relationship between helminth infections (helminthiasis) and allergic diseases. Although helminthiasis can cause immunosuppression, they can also stimulate a Th2-type immune response, characteristic of allergic diseases. These two effects seem antagonistic but can occur simultaneously [10]. In recent years, an increase in the prevalence of allergic diseases has been observed worldwide, including in our country. Particularly, food allergies are associated with considerable morbidity and mortality, representing a public health issue.

Antigens and Allergens of Anisakis simplex

The L3 and L4 larval stages of *A. simplex* include many antigenic components capable of inducing an immune response in the parasitized host, with expected variability related to both the parasite and the host [24]. In susceptible individuals, exposure to allergens can trigger allergic disease symptoms. IgE antibodies play a central role in the pathophysiology of these diseases. IgE binds to the high-affinity FcεRI receptor on mast cell and basophil membranes during the sensitization phase. In the effector phase of the allergic response, the presence of the allergen causes cross-linking, resulting in degranulation and the release of inflammatory mediators, leading to symptom manifestation (see Fig. 2.1) [25]. To date, 14 allergens of *Anisakis simplex* have been described (Table 2.1).

As previously mentioned, *A. simplex* extracts and their allergens show cross-reactivity with antigens from other sources, such as dust mites [26, 27], wasp venom [28], and cockroaches [29]. One of the allergens with the highest cross-reactivity is Anisakis tropomyosin (Ani s 3), which is phylogenetically related to that of crustaceans and insects and could explain the observed antibody reactivity [30]. In the case of cross-reactivity with wasp venom, it has been shown that allergic patients recognize carbohydrate epitopes present in Vespula [28].

Table 2.1 Allergens characterized in Anisakis

Allergen	Biochemical name	Molecular weight	Allergenicity	Reference
Ani s 1	Serine protease inhibitor-like	24 kDa	Of 49 *A. simplex*-sensitive patients, 68% showed IgE binding to Ani s 1 in immunoblotting	[31]
Ani s 2	Paramyosin	97 kDa	Of 26 *A. simplex*-sensitive patients, 23 (88%) showed IgE binding to purified Ani s 2 in ELISA assays	[32]
Ani s 3	Tropomyosin	41 kDa	8 of 62 patients with suspected *A. simplex* allergy (13%)	[33]
Ani s 4	Cysteine protease inhibitor	9 kDa	27% of sensitized subjects reacted to Ani s 4	[34]
Ani s 5	SXP/RAL-2 family protein	15 kDa	41 of 84 sera (49%) were positive in direct ELISA using recombinant protein	[35]
Ani s 6	Serine protease inhibitor	9.7 kDa	5 of 28 sera to *A. simplex* were positive in direct ELISA using recombinant protein	[36]
Ani s 7	Protein with unknown function	139 kDa	Ani s 7 was recognized by 92.9% and 92.5% of sera from patients with gastroallergic anisakiasis	[37]
Ani s 8	SXP/RAL-2 family protein	15 kDa	Of 28 patients allergic to *A. simplex*, 7 had IgE to purified Ani s 8 by ELISA	[38]
Ani s 9	SXP/RAL-2 family protein	14 kDa	5 of 36 patients allergic to *A. simplex* (13.8%) were positive to rAni s 9 and natural Ani s 9 by immunodetection	[39]
Ani s 10	Protein with unknown function	21 kDa	30 of 77 individuals allergic to *A. simplex* had IgE binding to recombinant Ani s 10 in non-reducing immunoblotting	[40]
Ani s 11	Protein with unknown function	27 kDa	14 of 30 sera from patients allergic to *A. simplex* showed IgE reactivity by fluorescence ELISA	[41]
Ani s 12	Protein with unknown function	31 kDa	17 of 30 sera from patients allergic to *A. simplex* showed IgE reactivity by fluorescence ELISA	[41]
Ani s 13	Hemoglobin	37 kDa	28 of 44 patients with gastroallergic anisakiasis had demonstrable IgE binding to the protein by hemoglobin-specific capture ELISA	[42]
Ani s 14	Third-stage larval protein with unknown function	24 kDa	14 of 26 patients reactive to *A. simplex* proteins tested positive in ELISA using purified recombinant allergen expressed in *E. coli*	[43]

Conclusions

The zoonotic infection caused by *A. simplex* is associated with a strong Th2-type response against excretory and somatic antigens of the parasite, which can cause a wide variety of clinical symptoms. The use of purified recombinant allergens of *A. simplex* and deglycosylated allergens increases the specificity and sensitivity of infection diagnosis, due to the high cross-reactivity that this parasite presents with other allergenic sources.

Lastly, the presence of these nematodes in fish poses a significant public health problem in societies that consume raw fish. Although raw fish consumption is not common in some countries, the globalization of traditional Japanese or Peruvian cuisine, with their iconic dishes (sushi and ceviches), can present a potential risk of new sensitizations in susceptible individuals. This is especially important considering that many of the fish consumed, for example in our country, are infected with parasites.

Glossary

Glossary of Acronyms

BAT Basophil Activation Test
ELISA Enzyme-Linked Immunosorbent Assay
FcεRI High-Affinity IgE Receptor
IgE Immunoglobulin E
L3 Third Larval Stage
WHO World Health Organization

Glossary of Terms

Anisakiasis An infection caused by consuming raw or undercooked fish containing larvae of the *Anisakis simplex* nematode.

Anisakis simplex A nematode from the Anisakidae family, known for causing foodborne infections and allergic reactions.

Allergen A substance that can cause an allergic reaction. *Anisakis simplex* has 14 known allergens.

Angioedema Swelling beneath the skin often caused by an allergic reaction, which can occur with *Anisakis simplex.*

Basophil Activation Test (BAT) A diagnostic test that measures basophil activation in response to allergens, useful for diagnosing Anisakis allergy.

Capture ELISA A laboratory technique used to detect and quantify substances, including deglycosylated specific allergens of *Anisakis simplex.*

Cross-reactivity When an allergen shares similar protein structures with another allergen, causing an immune response. Anisakis allergens can cross-react with dust mites, cockroaches, and wasp venom.

Deglycosylated Allergens Allergens that have had their carbohydrate portions removed to reduce cross-reactivity and improve diagnostic specificity.

Eosinophilic Gastroenteritis Inflammation of the stomach and intestines due to an accumulation of eosinophils, which can be triggered by *Anisakis simplex*.

Gastroallergic Anisakiasis A condition where ingestion of Anisakis larvae causes gastrointestinal symptoms and allergic reactions.

IgE (Immunoglobulin E) An antibody associated with allergic reactions. IgE-mediated responses are significant in *Anisakis simplex* allergies.

Intermediate Host An organism that harbors the larval or asexual stage of a parasite. Anisakis uses crustaceans and fish as intermediate hosts.

Larva The immature form of *Anisakis simplex*, particularly the third larval stage (L3) which infects humans.

Molecular Cloning A method used to create copies of DNA fragments, including those coding for Anisakis allergens.

Paramyosin A protein allergen from *Anisakis simplex* recognized by IgE antibodies in sensitized individuals.

Proteomic Profiling The study of the structure and function of proteins, including allergomes of *Anisakis simplex*.

Serine Protease Inhibitor A type of protein that can act as an allergen. *Anisakis simplex* has several serine protease inhibitor-like allergens.

Th2-Type Immune Response An immune response that involves Th2 cells and is characteristic of allergic reactions, often stimulated by *Anisakis simplex* infections.

Tropomyosin An allergen found in *Anisakis simplex* that shows cross-reactivity with crustaceans and insects.

Zoonotic Infection An infection that is transmissible from animals to humans, such as anisakiasis caused by *Anisakis simplex*.

Funding Part of Call 948 "Orquídeas, Women in Science 2024" supported by Minciencias through the Francisco José de Caldas Fund, project 109565, contract 112721-245-2024, Republic of Colombia.

References

1. Daschner A, Alonso-Gómez A, Cabañas R, Suarez-de-Parga JM, López-Serrano MC. Gastroallergic anisakiasis: borderline between food allergy and parasitic disease-clinical and allergologic evaluation of 20 patients with confirmed acute parasitism by Anisakis simplex. J Allergy Clin Immunol enero de. 2000;105(1 Pt 1):176–81.
2. Packi K, Rudek A, Matysiak J, Klimczak S, Matuszewska E, Rzetecka N, et al. Food allergies and parasites in children. Foods enero de. 2023;12(13):2465.
3. Moreno-Ancillo A, Caballero MT, Cabañas R, Contreras J, Martin-Barroso JA, Barranco P, et al. Allergic reactions to Anisakis simplex parasitizing seafood. Ann Allergy Asthma Immunol. 1 de septiembre de. 1997;79(3):246–50.
4. del Pozo V, Arrieta I, Tuñon T, Cortegano I, Gomez B, Cárdaba B, et al. Immunopathogenesis of human gastrointestinal infection by Anisakis simplex. J Allergy Clin Immunol septiembre de. 1999;104(3 Pt 1):637–43.
5. Golden O, Araújo AC, Caldeira AJR, Santos MJ. Raw fish consumption in Portugal: Commonly consumed fish species and associated risk factors for anisakiosis. Food Control. 1 de marzo de. 2023;145:109457.

6. Domingo-Hernández AM, Morales-Yuste M, Buzo-Domínguez S, Adroher FJ, Benítez R. Anisakis infection in anchovies (Engraulis encrasicolus) from Iberian waters, southwestern Europe: post-mortem larval migration. Res Vet Sci 1 de abril de. 2023;157:26–34.
7. Baird FJ, Gasser RB, Jabbar A, Lopata AL. Foodborne anisakiasis and allergy. Mol Cell Probes. 1 de agosto de. 2014;28(4):167–74.
8. Lucas D, Greta G, Bygvraa DA, Canals ML, Adam B, Lux H, et al. Occupational allergic diseases among harvesting fishermen on the open sea: a systematic review. Ann Allergy Asthma Immunol [Internet]. 26 de abril de 2023 [citado 30 de junio de 2023]; Disponible en; 2023. https://www.sciencedirect.com/science/article/pii/S1081120623002855
9. Nieuwenhuizen NE, Lopata AL. Allergic reactions to Anisakis found in fish. Curr Allergy Asthma Rep 20 de julio de. 2014;14(8):455.
10. Audicana MT. Anisakis, something is moving inside the fish. Pathogens. marzo de. 2022;11(3):326.
11. Villafruela Cives M, Henríquez SA. Anisakiasis. Rev Esp Enfermedades Dig marzo de. 2010;102(3):216–6.
12. Pichler WJ. Anisakiasis: immunity, allergy or both? Lessons on the natural role of immunoglobulin E from a nematode infestation. Clin Exp Allergy J Br Soc Allergy Clin Immunol. septiembre de. 1999;29(9):1161–3.
13. Viñas M, Postigo I, Suñén E, Martínez J. Urticaria and silent parasitism by Ascaridoidea: Component-resolved diagnosis reinforces the significance of this association. PLoS Negl Trop Dis. 3 de abril de. 2020;14(4):e0008177.
14. Carballeda-Sangiao N, Sánchez-Alonso I, Navas A, Arcos SC, de Palencia PF, Careche M, et al. Anisakis simplex products impair intestinal epithelial barrier function and occludin and zonula occludens-1 localisation in differentiated Caco-2 cells. PLoS Negl Trop Dis. 6 de julio de. 2020;14(7):e0008462.
15. Pontone M, Giovannini M, Barni S, Mori F, Venturini E, Galli L, et al. IgE-mediated Anisakis allergy in children. Allergol Immunopathol (Madr). 1 de enero de. 2023;51(1):98–109.
16. Ramos L, Alonso C, Guilarte M, Vilaseca J, Santos J, Malagelada JR. Anisakis simplex-induced small bowel obstruction after fish ingestion: preliminary evidence for response to parenteral corticosteroids. Clin Gastroenterol Hepatol. 1 de julio de. 2005;3(7):667–71.
17. Filauro M, Rollandi GA, Cassola G, Quilici P, Angelini G, Belli F, et al. Gastrointestinal bleeding due to suspected anisakiasis: challenging differential diagnosis for a rare disease. Updat Surg. 1 de septiembre de. 2011;63(3):213–7.
18. Lorenzo S, Iglesias R, Leiro J, Ubeira FM, Ansotegui I, García M, et al. Usefulness of currently available methods for the diagnosis of Anisakis simplex allergy. Allergy. 2000;55(7):627–33.
19. Brusca I, Barrale M, Zarcone M, Fruscione S, Onida R, De Bella DD, et al. Basophil activation test in the diagnosis of Anisakis allergy: an observational study from an area of high seafood consumption in Italy. Pathogens junio de. 2023;12(6):777.
20. de Las Vecillas L, Muñoz-Cacho P, López-Hoyos M, Monttecchiani V, Martínez-Sernández V, Ubeira FM, et al. Analysis of Ani s 7 and Ani s 1 allergens as biomarkers of sensitization and allergy severity in human anisakiasis. Sci Rep. 9 de julio de. 2020;10(1):11275.
21. Rahmati AR, Kiani B, Afshari A, Moghaddas E, Williams M, Shamsi S. World-wide prevalence of Anisakis larvae in fish and its relationship to human allergic anisakiasis: a systematic review. Parasitol Res. 1 de noviembre de. 2020;119(11):3585–94.
22. Otsubo S, Nishiyama T, Okada N, Ando Y, Yamada K, Maeda Y, et al. Ventricular fibrillation by anaphylaxis following consumption of blue_skinned fish: anaphylactic shock due to anisakis allergy. Acute Med Surg. abril de. 2016;3(2):159–62.
23. Aibinu IE, Smooker PM, Lopata AL. Anisakis Nematodes in Fish and Shellfish- from infection to allergies. Int J Parasitol Parasites Wildl. 1 de agosto de. 2019;9:384–93.
24. Kochanowski M, Dąbrowska J, Różycki M, Karamon J, Sroka J, Cencek T. Proteomic profiling reveals new insights into the allergomes of anisakis simplex, pseudoterranova decipiens, and Contracaecum osculatum. J Parasitol. 8 de septiembre de. 2020;106(5):572–88.
25. Dramburg S, Hilger C, Santos AF, de las Vecillas L, Aalberse RC, Acevedo N, et al. EAACI molecular allergology user's guide 2.0. Pediatr Allergy Immunol. 2023;34(S28):e13854.

26. Johansson E, Aponno M, Lundberg M, Van Hage-Hamsten M. Allergenic cross-reactivity between the nematode Anisakis simplex and the dust mites Acarus siro, Lepidoglyphus destructor, Tyrophagus putrescentiae, and Dermatophagoides pteronyssinus. Allergy. 2001;56(7):660–6.
27. Bernardini R, Mistrello G, Novembre E, Roncarolo D, Zanotta S, Lombardi E, et al. Cross-Reactivity between IgE-Binding Proteins from Anisakis Simplex and Dermatophagoides Pteronyssinus. Int J Immunopathol Pharmacol. 1 de octubre de. 2005;18(4):671–5.
28. Rodríguez-Pérez R, Monsalve RI, Galán A, Perez-Piñar T, Umpierrez A, Lluch-Bernal M, et al. Cross-reactivity between Anisakis spp. and Wasp Venom Allergens. Int Arch Allergy Immunol. 13 de febrero de. 2014;163(3):179–84.
29. Pascual CY, Crespo JF, Martin SS, Ornia N, Ortega N, Caballero T, et al. Cross-reactivity between IgE-binding proteins from Anisakis German cockroach, and chironomids. Allergy. 1997;52(5):514–20.
30. Kamath SD, Abdel Rahman AM, Komoda T, Lopata AL. Impact of heat processing on the detection of the major shellfish allergen tropomyosin in crustaceans and molluscs using specific monoclonal antibodies. Food Chem 15 de diciembre de. 2013;141(4):4031–9.
31. Moneo I, Caballero ML, Gómez F, Ortega E, Alonso MJ. Isolation and characterization of a major allergen from the fish parasite Anisakis simplex. J Allergy Clin Immunol julio de. 2000;106(1 Pt 1):177–82.
32. Pérez-Pérez J, Fernández-Caldas E, Marañón F, Sastre J, Bernal ML, Rodríguez J, et al. Molecular cloning of paramyosin, a new allergen of Anisakis simplex. Int Arch Allergy Immunol. octubre de. 2000;123(2):120–9.
33. Asturias JA, Eraso E, Moneo I, Martínez A. Is tropomyosin an allergen in Anisakis? Allergy. septiembre de. 2000;55(9):898–9.
34. Moneo I, Caballero ML, González-Muñoz M, Rodríguez-Mahillo AI, Rodríguez-Perez R, Silva A. Isolation of a heat-resistant allergen from the fish parasite Anisakis simplex. Parasitol Res julio de. 2005;96(5):285–9.
35. Caballero ML, Moneo I, Gómez-Aguado F, Corcuera MT, Casado I, Rodríguez-Pérez R. Isolation of Ani s 5, an excretory-secretory and highly heat-resistant allergen useful for the diagnosis of Anisakis larvae sensitization. Parasitol Res. octubre de. 2008;103(5):1231–3.
36. Kobayashi Y, Ishizaki S, Shimakura K, Nagashima Y, Shiomi K. Molecular cloning and expression of two new allergens from Anisakis simplex. Parasitol Res. mayo de. 2007;100(6):1233–41.
37. Cuéllar C, Daschner A, Valls A, De Frutos C, Fernández-Fígares V, Anadón AM, et al. Ani s 1 and Ani s 7 recombinant allergens are able to differentiate distinct Anisakissimplex-associated allergic clinical disorders. Arch Dermatol Res. 1 de mayo de. 2012;304(4):283–8.
38. Kobayashi Y, Shimakura K, Ishizaki S, Nagashima Y, Shiomi K. Purification and cDNA cloning of a new heat-stable allergen from Anisakis simplex. Mol Biochem Parasitol. octubre de. 2007;155(2):138–45.
39. Rodriguez-Perez R, Moneo I, Rodriguez-Mahillo A, Caballero ML. Cloning and expression of Ani s 9, a new Anisakis simplex allergen. Mol Biochem Parasitol. junio de. 2008;159(2):92–7.
40. Caballero ML, Umpierrez A, Moneo I, Rodriguez-Perez R. Ani s 10, a new Anisakis simplex allergen: cloning and heterologous expression. Parasitol Int. junio de. 2011;60(2):209–12.
41. Kobayashi Y, Ohsaki K, Ikeda K, Kakemoto S, Ishizaki S, Shimakura K, et al. Identification of novel three allergens from Anisakis simplex by chemiluminescent immunoscreening of an expression cDNA library. Parasitol Int. 1 de junio de. 2011;60(2):144–50.
42. González-Fernández J, Daschner A, Nieuwenhuizen NE, Lopata AL, Frutos CD, Valls A, et al. Haemoglobin, a new major allergen of Anisakis simplex. Int J Parasitol. mayo de. 2015;45(6):399–407.
43. Kobayashi Y, Kakemoto S, Shimakura K, Shiomi K. Molecular cloning and expression of a new major allergen, Ani s 14, from Anisakis simplex. Shokuhin Eiseigaku Zasshi J Food Hyg Soc Jpn. 2015;56(5):194–9.

Chapter 3
Allergy, Intolerance, and Intoxication to Dairy Products: Milk

Albeiro Marrugo Padilla, Erika Rodríguez Cavallo, Darío Mendez Cuadro, and Nathalia Villadiego Portacio

Introduction

Adverse food reactions (AFRs) are common worldwide; they have significantly increased over the past decade. They are considered a serious health problem due to their clinical impact, economic burden, and effect on patient's quality of life [1]. According to the AAAAI and the EAACI Nomenclature Committee, AFRs are any abnormal clinical response attributed to the ingestion, contact, or inhalation of food, its derivatives, or an additive, with mechanisms that may or may not have an immunological component [1–3]. The prevalence of AFRs in adults worldwide exceeds 30% and can surprisingly reach up to 90% when focusing solely on food intolerance, with lactose intolerance being the most common [3].

The prognosis and clinical manifestations of AFRs depend on the underlying etiology and the pathophysiological processes involved. AFRs are classified as

A. M. Padilla (✉)
TOXSA Research Group, Faculty of Health Cartagena, Corporación Universitaria Rafael Núñez, Cartagena, Colombia
e-mail: albeiro.marrugo@curnvirtual.edu.co

E. R. Cavallo
Faculty of Pharmaceutical Sciences, Analytical Chemistry and Biomedicine Group, University of Cartagena, Cartagena, Bolívar, Colombia
e-mail: erodriguezc1@unicartagena.edu.co

D. M. Cuadro
Faculty of Exact and Natural Sciences, Analytical Chemistry and Biomedicine Group, University of Cartagena, Cartagena, Colombia
e-mail: dmendezc@unicartagena.edu.co

N. V. Portacio
Corporación Universitaria Rafael Núñez, Cartagena, Bolívar, Colombia
e-mail: nvilladiegop10@curnvirtual.edu.co

M. G. Múnera Gómez et al. (eds.), *Allergies, Poisoning and Intolerance to Common Substances*, https://doi.org/10.1007/978-3-031-93658-6_3

toxic and nontoxic reactions. Toxic reactions are independent of the food components and result from the presence of chemical contaminants (xenobiotics) such as pesticides, antibiotics, and hormones in the food, the presence of pathogens like *Campylobacter jejuni*, *Escherichia coli*, *Listeria monocytogenes*, and toxins produced by microorganisms (e.g., enterotoxins of Staphylococcus aureus) [4]. Nontoxic adverse food reactions, on the other hand, are contingent upon the inherent components of the food and encompass sensitivities (immune-mediated reactions) and intolerances (nonimmune-mediated reactions), distinguished by whether they trigger an immune response or involve a mechanical alteration [1–3]. In this chapter, we will focus on adverse reactions arising from the consumption of cow's milk and its derivatives.

Nontoxic Adverse Reactions to Bovine Milk

Bovine Milk Allergy

Bovine milk allergy (BMA), also known as Cow's Milk Protein Allergy (CMPA), and APLV (Allergy to Proteins of Cow's Milk) is the most common pediatric allergic disease globally, affecting 2–6% of children, especially during the first year of life. It is a nontoxic adverse reaction resulting from the consumption of cow's milk and its derivatives, accounting for 10–40% of all food allergies [5]. This condition represents a hypersensitivity reaction to milk proteins, specifically caseins (CAS) and bovine β-lactoglobulin (β-Lg), which are among the initial allergens infants encounter during the transition from breastfeeding to infant formulas or direct consumption of cow's milk [6, 7]. BMA usually resolves in most cases before adulthood but can also occur later in life [8].

The clinical manifestations of BMA change depending on the type of immune reaction (IgE-mediated, non-IgE-mediated, or mixed) and the affected organ: skin (50–70%), gastrointestinal tract (50–60%), and respiratory system (20–30%). Factors that increase the risk of developing BMA include genetic predisposition, early intake of lesser amounts of cow's milk protein (CMP), and gut microbiome-related factors [9].

The earliest documented adverse reactions to bovine milk allergy (BMA) can be traced back to Hippocrates (before 370 B.C.). Approximately 500 years later, Galen of Pergamon, a renowned Greek physician and researcher, conducted a correlational study on symptoms associated with milk consumption as described by Hippocrates [10]. In the early twentieth century, there was a notable increase in observations of adverse reactions to cow's milk protein (CMP). Today, cow's milk remains one of the first foods introduced into an infant's diet and thus stands as one of the primary and earliest causes of food allergy in early childhood [6, 7, 11].

BMA has an annual incidence of 2–3% (though incidences of up to 7.5% have been reported) and peaks during early childhood to decrease with age [12–14]. Its prevalence differs significantly between studies, attributable to different diagnostic methods, variations in the age groups studied, geographic factors, etc. Its prevalence is higher in preschool children (0.6–2.5%) compared to older children, adolescents (0.5%), and adults (less than 0.3%) [15]. Over the past decade, the prevalence of BMA has increased significantly due to industrialization, cultural changes, and the working dynamics of breastfeeding mothers, leading to reduced breastfeeding duration and increased use of cow's milk-based infant formulas. Bovine milk proteins are among the eight major food allergens; in 2021, a new food joined the list of major allergens, turning "The Big 8" into "The Big 9." They are eggs, soybean, wheat, peanuts, tree nuts, fish, shellfish, and sesame [6, 8].

Cow's Milk Allergens

Proteins from bovine milk (*Bos domesticus*) are included in the official list of allergens issued by the World Health Organization [16]. Currently, more than 40 types of proteins have been characterized in this food, with over 20 antigens like those in the human species identified. All milk proteins are considered high quality due to their high essential amino acid content, corrected chemical score, bioavailability, and good digestibility [17–19]. The most important milk proteins produced in the cow's mammary gland include α-lactalbumin and β-lactoglobulin, the main components of serum protein (~20%), along with caseins (~80%). Additionally, other proteins such as bovine serum albumin, lactoferrin, and immunoglobulins originated from blood [8, 20]. Caseins are the insoluble fraction, while whey proteins (WPs) are dissolved in the milk matrix [17–19]. Both groups have been shown to induce hypersensitivity reactions; however, caseins are considered the primary allergens of bovine milk [21–25].

Bovine milk allergy (BMA) is a condition associated with the introduction of artificial feeding in infancy. One explanation for the immunoreactivity associated with cow's milk (CM) ingestion is the quantitative differences in its protein content compared to human breast milk (HBM). In this context, the protein content in CM is three times higher than in HBM, and the balance between WPs and caseins is 20:80, while in HBM, it is 60:40. Additionally, HBM lacks β-lactoglobulin, the proportion of αs1-casein is very low, and β-casein has a different phosphorylation profile and a generally lower degree of phosphorylation than its counterpart in CM [26, 27].

Caseins

Caseins constitute the predominant protein fraction in bovine milk, accounting for approximately 80% of its total mass. These proteins are classified under the general designation (Bos d 8) according to the official WHO allergen list, with specific components identified by different codes: Bos d 9 (αS1-casein), Bos d 10 (αS2-casein), Bos d 11 (β-casein), and Bos d 12 (κ-casein) [16].

Structurally, caseins are secretory phosphoproteins organized in micellar formations capable of binding polyvalent cations such as calcium through their phosphate groups. This structural feature underpins their biological functions, which include roles in secretion, digestion, and nutrient absorption [28]. αS1-casein is a phosphoprotein with a molecular weight of 23 kDa, characterized by a high content of proline residues. This protein is absent in human milk, which is the main reason for its high immunogenicity. Approximately 50% of serum samples from patients with cow's milk allergy react with this casein. Epitope mapping studies have identified various IgE recognition sites (IgE-binding epitopes), which are linear and primarily located at the carboxyl-terminal end of the protein (residues 181–199) [16, 20]. However, different IgE epitopes were mapped throughout this protein. Chatchatee et al. (2001) identified two IgE-binding sites (residues 69–78 and 173–194), which are recognized by most patients over nine years old with persistent allergy [29], while Cerecedo et al. (2008) identified one in the region of 28–50, which is 75% reactive to IgE [30].

Another allergenic casein is αS2-casein, which consists of 207 amino acids and has a molecular mass of 25.2 kDa. According to epidemiological studies, the prevalence of sensitization to this protein in allergic patients is 90%. To date, more than six IgE-binding epitopes have been identified. Cerecedo et al. (2008) identified seven regions, with the most reactive being between amino acids 1–20, 13–32, 67–86, and 181–207 [30]. β-casein and κ-casein have less immunological reactivity compared to the proteins described above [5, 31]. Chatchatee et al. (2001) identified six major and three secondary IgE-binding epitopes in β-casein, as well as eight major and one secondary IgG-binding regions. In κ-casein, eight major IgE-binding epitopes were detected, along with two major and two secondary IgG-binding epitopes [32].

Whey Proteins

Whey proteins (WPs) represent approximately 20% of the total protein mass in bovine milk. This group includes β-lactoglobulin (β-Lg) and α-lactalbumin (α-La) as the main components. In smaller proportions, it also contains immunoglobulins, bovine serum albumin, lactoferrin, lactoperoxidase, and lysozymes, among others [33, 34]. WPs provide essential amino acids and regulate functions related to immunity and fatty acid transport. Among these, β-Lg (Bos d 5) is the most abundant, constituting 51% of the total WPs. This globular protein has 162 amino acid residues (including more than 20 essential amino acids), a molecular weight of 18 kDa, and plays a role in the transport of lipid molecules such as retinol [35]. Allergies associated with β-Lg can affect up to 80% of the population [20].

α-La (Bos d 4) is a less allergenic protein than β-Lg, comprising 22% of the WP fraction. It consists of 123 amino acid residues and has a molecular weight of 14.2 kDa. This protein is involved in lactose synthesis and the transport of metals such as cobalt, magnesium, and zinc [20]. WPs are primary allergens in children, including α-La and β-Lg, whereas in adolescents and adults, the casein fraction is more allergenic [(αS1-casein (32%), αS2-casein (10%), β-casein (28%), and κ-casein (10%)], with αS1-casein being the most important allergen in this fraction [6, 22, 36–38].

Pathophysiology of Cow's Milk Allergy

The allergenic process mediated by cow's milk proteins (CMP) occurs in the gastrointestinal tract; however, in some susceptible individuals, the skin also plays a significant role in promoting allergic events. After ingestion, CMPs are destroyed by gastric acid and digestive enzymes in the stomach and intestines (caseins are more susceptible to digestion, while WPs may reach the small intestine intact). The remaining proteins and peptides are transported from the intestinal mucosa's lumen to the lamina propria through specialized epithelial cells (M cells) located over Peyer's patches.

Another well-characterized route for allergen transport to the lamina propria is through dendritic cells (DCs), which can extend their dendrites into the intestinal lumen to capture proteins and peptides. Once the antigen is captured, the DC internalizes, processes, and presents it to naive T lymphocytes in the draining areas of the T cells in the lymph nodes via their MHC class II molecules. The activation of different DC subsets, and the expression of co-stimulatory molecules are important for determining the subsequent immune response (Fig. 3.1) [10, 39].

Three mechanisms are associated with the pathophysiology and clinical signs and symptoms of CMP allergy. The first is an IgE-mediated reaction (whose symptoms occur immediately after consuming the allergen or a few minutes after exposure). The second mechanism involves non-IgE-mediated reactions (delayed reactions with symptoms occurring hours or days after allergen exposure). Finally, the third mechanism combines IgE-mediated and non-IgE-mediated mechanisms [40]. IgE-mediated CMP allergy (type I hypersensitivity or anaphylactic reactions) accounts for approximately 65% of adverse reactions induced by CMP.

Clinical symptoms result in local skin conditions such as urticaria, rashes, oral allergy syndrome, facial angioedema, respiratory system issues, and gastrointestinal tract disturbances; in severe cases, it presents as systemic anaphylactic reactions [7]. The process begins with antigen-presenting cells processing the allergen (caseins, α-La, or β-Lg), promoting the activation of a naive T lymphocyte into a helper type 2 (TH2). TH2 lymphocytes and the cytokines

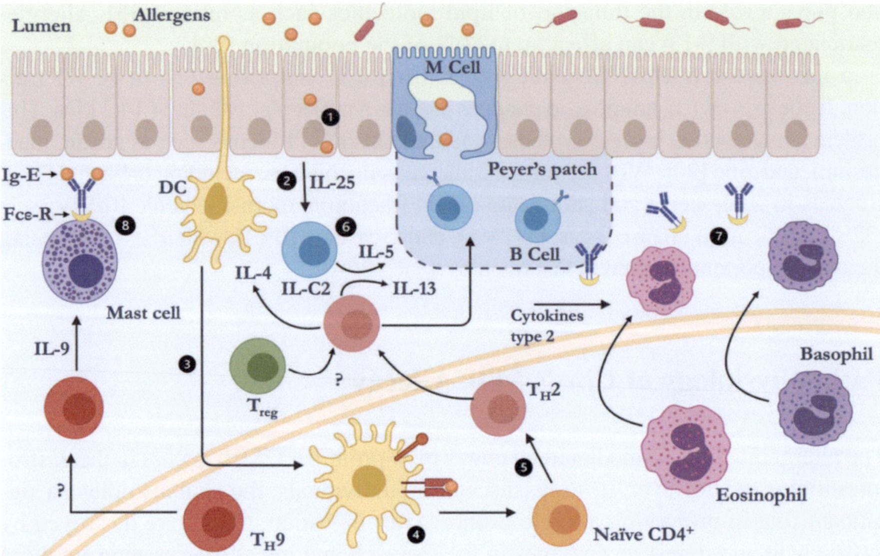

Fig. 3.1 The figure illustrates the immune response to allergens in the intestine. Allergens pass through M cells into the Peyer's patches, where dendritic cells present antigens to naive T cells. These differentiate into TH2 and TH9 cells, promoting the release of cytokines such as IL-4, IL-5, and IL-9, which activate ILC2 cells, eosinophils, and basophils. Mast cells are activated by IgE, releasing inflammatory mediators that contribute to the allergic response

associated with the process stimulate the proliferation of B cells, promoting isotype class switch recombination to IgE and differentiation into antibody-secreting plasma cells. Released IgE mediated immediate phase reactions by inducing mast cell and basophil degranulation. Upon subsequent exposure to the allergen, it binds to serum IgE molecules. The cross-linked complex is recognized by mast cells and basophils, causing degranulation and release of chemical mediators, including histamine, responsible for the wide variety of clinical manifestations observed with immediate reactions, which can be limited to a single organ or multisystemic, causing anaphylaxis [10, 39].

Non-IgE-mediated CMP allergy is a type IV hypersensitivity reaction orchestrated by delayed-type hypersensitivity cells, typically presenting as gastrointestinal symptoms [7]. This occurs when TH1 cells activate macrophages after recognizing allergens to produce lytic enzymes and cytotoxic T cells (CD8+), which directly attack host cells, causing inflammation and tissue damage, mainly due to lysosomal enzymes, reactive oxygen species, nitric oxide, and pro-inflammatory cytokines secreted by activated macrophages. Non-IgE-mediated allergies are less well-known than type I hypersensitivity reactions and are believed to involve other antibody-mediated mechanisms as well [41, 42]. Finally, mixed CMP allergies are characterized by both IgE-dependent and independent mechanisms. Clinical manifestations derived from IgE-independent factors include atopic dermatitis associated with late-onset food allergy (6–48 h after exposure) caused by TH2 cell action and eosinophilic gastrointestinal disorders, often triggered by milk allergens and caused by eosinophilic infiltration of tissues [43].

Diagnosis of Cow's Milk Allergy

To achieve an accurate diagnosis of cow's milk allergy (CMA), it is necessary to conduct a detailed patient history, including age, onset of symptoms, frequency of occurrence, time of appearance after allergen ingestion, and family history of atopy. For patients who are breastfeeding, it is crucial to characterize the mother's diet, particularly her consumption of dairy products. It is important to note that none of the routine clinical diagnostic tests can generate a precise diagnosis of CMA. Skin prick tests, specific IgE determination, and patch tests only indicate sensitization to the substrate without confirming an allergic reaction. The non-specificity of clinical manifestations associated with CMA often leads to diagnostic failures. The double-blind, placebo-controlled food challenge is considered the gold standard for diagnosing CMA, but in practice, an open challenge is usually performed. Unfortunately, this process is costly, requires extensive preparation, is time-consuming, and is difficult to carry out in some places [7].

The diagnosis of CMA involves an elimination diet excluding the allergen for two to four weeks, followed by a challenge with CMP. Currently, there is a Cow's Milk-related Symptom Score (CoMiSS®) (Table 3.1) to facilitate the diagnosis

Table 3.1 CoMiSS®: cow's milk-related symptom score

Symptom	Score range	Description
Regurgitation	0–9	Frequency and volume of regurgitation episodes
Stool consistency	0–9	Frequency and consistency of stools, including diarrhea or constipation
Skin symptoms	0–6	Presence and severity of eczema and urticaria
Respiratory symptoms	0–3	Presence and severity of respiratory symptoms such as wheezing or cough
Crying time	0–6	Duration and frequency of crying episodes, indicative of discomfort or pain
Total score	0–33	Sum of all individual scores, indicating the overall impact of cow's milk consumption on the patient's symptoms

process in infants. This is a simple, quick, and easy-to-use tool that aids in early diagnosis. It includes gastrointestinal manifestations (regurgitation and altered defecation), skin signs (eczema and urticaria), respiratory tract symptoms, and general symptoms such as crying time. The CoMiSS ranges from 0 to 33 points, from the absence of symptoms and signs to multiple manifestations and degrees of severity [44–46]. CoMiSS has been shown to have a sensitivity of 87.5% and a specificity of 78.6% [7].

IgE-Mediated Tests

The measurement of specific IgE in blood samples and skin prick tests can establish a patient's sensitization to cow's milk proteins (CMP). The probability of a positive result in a controlled oral food challenge exceeds 95% when the specific IgE concentration is greater than 1 IU/mL in children under two years of age and when it is greater than 15 IU/mL in older children [7]. Quantifying the results of these two tests helps predict the likelihood of an additional reaction and is therefore useful for establishing prognosis: the higher the antibody titer, the greater the severity of the reaction. Children with gastrointestinal manifestations associated with CMA are more likely to have negative specific IgE test results compared to patients with skin manifestations [47, 48].

Skin prick tests are used to detect the presence of IgE antibodies bound to tissue; however, a positive result does not confirm an allergy. A wheal size of ≥5 mm is associated with greater specificity. A negative skin test rules out IgE-mediated reactions, with negative predictive values of 95%. The wheal size is significantly larger in children with the persistent disease compared to those who outgrow CMA and is therefore useful as a prognostic indicator. Infants generally respond less to skin prick tests [48].

Specific IgG Antibodies and Other Nonstandardized Tests and Procedures

The determination of IgG antibodies against CMP has no role in diagnosing this pathology, until now or it could be more relevant in non-IgE mediated CMA. Other alternatives include evaluating basophil histamine release/activation, lymphocyte stimulation, mediator release assays, and endoscopic allergen provocation, which are used as research protocols but not in clinical practice. In patients with significant and persistent gastrointestinal symptoms, upper and/or lower endoscopies with multiple biopsies are appropriate; however, macroscopic lesions and histological findings, such as mucosal atrophy or eosinophilic infiltrates, are neither sensitive nor specific for CMA [47, 48].

Clinical Management and Therapeutic Options

The safest strategy for the treatment or management of CMA is to avoid consuming allergenic food. The decision to use a substitute formula to meet the patient's nutritional needs should be based on age and any history of other food allergies. For infants exclusively breastfed, elimination involves excluding dairy products from the mother's diet. Mothers need to receive calcium supplements and dietary advice to avoid nutritional deficiencies. All cow's milk-based formulas and complementary foods containing its derivatives should be avoided in exclusively breastfed infants. On the other hand, extensively hydrolyzed formulas (EHF) and amino acid-based formulas are the two most used alternatives for patients not receiving breast milk or those not improving with exclusive breastfeeding and cow's milk elimination [7].

EHF and amino acid-based formulas are defined as foods with hydrolyzed proteins of animal (caseins or WPs) or vegetable (soy) origin that possess reduced allergenicity and are well tolerated by at least 90% of children with CMA, with a 95% confidence interval, when administered prospectively, randomized, double-blind, and placebo-controlled in clinical trials [49].

Intolerance to Bovine Milk

Bovine milk intolerance is one of the most common nonimmune-mediated AFRs worldwide, capable of affecting all age groups. This condition can be described as an intestinal mucosa disorder in which the patient presents alterations in the digestion and absorption of lactose ("milk sugar"), due to a reduced or absent activity of the enzyme lactase or reduced or absent synthesis of this enzyme [50, 51].

Lactose is a disaccharide composed of the monosaccharides D-galactose and D-glucose via a β-1,4 glycosidic bond found in the milk of mammals such as humans, cows, sheep, goats, and buffaloes, with concentrations of 7.0 mg/100 mL, 4.7–5.0 mg/100 mL, 4.4–4.8 mg/100 mL, 4.2–4.8 mg/100 mL, and 4.8–5.0 mg/100 mL, respectively. For proper utilization, lactose must be hydrolyzed into its constituent monosaccharides, a process catalyzed by the enzyme lactase-phlorizin hydrolase (lactase) present in the enterocytes of the intestinal mucosa, especially in the mid-jejunum [50, 51].

The ability to digest lactose during infancy is crucial for the growth and survival of the newborn. Generally, a term baby can digest between 60 and 70 g of lactose per day, equivalent to one liter of breast milk [52]. Studies have shown that congenital lactase deficiency is fatal if not diagnosed shortly after birth. Once released, glucose and galactose are absorbed by active transport in the intestine via the sodium/glucose cotransporter 1 (SGLT-1), a protein located in the enterocyte membrane, which co-transports glucose or galactose and two sodium ions (Na+) from the intestinal lumen to the cytoplasm of these cells. Subsequently, the monosaccharides are transferred from the cytosol to the blood by the transporter (GLUT-2), present on the other side of the enterocyte membrane. Glucose is used as an energy source, while galactose is converted into glucose or used as a component of glycolipids and glycoproteins [51]. A small amount of lactose may reach the colon undigested, where it is fermented by local microbiota microorganisms, producing short-chain fatty acids (butyric acid, propionic acid, acetic acid) in a process known as colonic carbohydrate salvage [50].

There is an evolutionarily conserved normal pattern of lactase production, which begins in fetal life (eighth week of gestation) and reaches a maximum of around six months of age, progressively decreasing until it is completely lost a few years after weaning [4]. This reduction in lactase (also mistakenly called lactase deficiency) occurs in approximately 75% of adult humans, leading to poor lactose digestion and the appearance of gastrointestinal symptoms [52, 53].

Lactose intolerance (LI) is a highly prevalent condition worldwide, with clinical manifestations that can be confused with other conditions such as celiac disease, bacterial overgrowth syndrome, or irritable bowel syndrome (functional gastrointestinal disorders). According to epidemiological studies, the prevalence of confirmed cases of LI worldwide ranges from 57%, with percentages of 15%, 50%, 70%, and 100% in Europe, America, Asia, and Africa, respectively [3, 51, 54].

Pathophysiology of Lactose Intolerance

Lactose intolerance (LI) is characterized by the accumulation of disaccharides in the intestine due to disruptions in digestion and absorption processes [55]. LI manifests in four main forms: congenital, neonatal, primary lactase deficiency, and secondary lactase deficiency, each distinguished by the underlying causes of reduced intestinal lactase levels and associated symptoms from undigested lactose in the colon [56, 57].

Congenital Lactase Deficiency (CLD): Also known as congenital alactasia, this is an extremely rare and severe autosomal recessive genetic disorder that disturbs the functional capacity of the intestinal protein lactase-phlorizin hydrolase (LPH) caused by mutations in the gene encoding lactase (LCT gene) located chromosome 2 (2q21). After birth, due to the inability to digest lactose, the major carbohydrate in mammalian milk leads to severe symptoms such as diarrhea, acidosis, hypercalcemia, and nephrocalcinosis, which are potentially life threatening [56–58].

Primary Lactase Deficiency

Primary lactase deficiency, also referred to as acquired hypolactasia or adult-type hypolactasia, is characterized by a significant reduction in lactase activity, often exceeding 95%. This condition represents the most prevalent cause of lactose intolerance (LI) worldwide, with an estimated prevalence of approximately 75%.

Primary lactase deficiency typically manifests after weaning, between the ages of 3 and 5. It is important to note that lactose malabsorption is not classified as a disease but rather as a normal physiological pattern observed in mammals.

Lactase persistence is inherited as a highly penetrant autosomal dominant trait [4, 53, 56]. The most common mechanism for lactase persistence is genetic polymorphism, involving a single nucleotide substitution on chromosome 2 that affects the lactase gene (LCT). Specifically, at least three polymorphic variants regulate LCT gene expression. The substitution of thymine for cytosine at position 13910 (SNP C/T-13910) is associated with lactase persistence, whereas the homozygous C/C-13910 genotype is linked to lactase nonpersistence [54].

Secondary lactase deficiency is a transient condition resulting from physical damage to the small intestine lining due to medications, infections, diseases, surgical procedures, or radiotherapy affecting enterocytes. It is particularly clinically significant in children, especially in regions with high incidences of disease and malnutrition [4, 53, 56].

LI occurs when the intestinal lactose load exceeds the capacity of available enzymatic activity. Fermentation of excess lactose by colonic microflora yields short-chain fatty acids, predominantly acetate, along with significant quantities of hydrogen, methane, and carbon dioxide. These gases increase intestinal transit time and intracolonic pressure, leading to symptoms such as abdominal pain, distension, flatulence, and visceral cramps. Furthermore, unabsorbed lactose creates an osmotic load that draws electrolytes and water into the intestinal lumen, potentially causing rapid transit and loose stools [4, 51, 53, 54, 56]. Microbial production of lactic acid further exacerbates osmotic effects, contributing to diarrhea [50], while excessive methane production can lead to constipation in some cases [54]. Symptoms of LI generally appear when lactase activity drops below 50%. These symptoms usually occur 30 min to 2 h after consuming lactose-containing foods and are like those of other enzymatic deficiencies. They include intestinal noises, distension, abdominal spasms localized in a periumbilical region or lower quadrant, flatulence, voluminous and frothy diarrhea (in some cases, constipation), abdominal gurgling, nausea, and vomiting.

LI much less frequently causes extraintestinal symptoms such as headaches, dizziness, short-term memory loss, intense fatigue, muscle pain, and arthralgia. The intensity and duration of symptoms vary depending on factors such as individual susceptibility, pathological conditions (comorbidities like irritable bowel syndrome, Crohn's disease, colitis, which can exacerbate symptoms), and the amount of lactose ingested [50, 51].

In addition to the symptoms described above, patients with LI may also experience extraintestinal symptoms such as memory impairment, headaches, musculoskeletal pain, cardiac rhythm disorders, depression, anxiety, oral mucosal ulcers, menstrual cycle disturbances, eczema, allergic base pathologies (sinusitis, rhinitis, asthma), acne, and increased urination frequency. These disorders can be caused by the excessive production of chemical compounds derived from the fermentation process (acetone, acetaldehyde, ethanol, peptides) [51].

Diagnosis of Lactose Intolerance

Currently, several diagnostic methods for lactose intolerance (LI) are divided into invasive and noninvasive categories. Invasive methods include genetic tests and the determination of lactase activity in intestinal mucosa fragments obtained via biopsy. Noninvasive methods, such as measuring hydrogen in exhaled breath (currently considered the test of choice), glucose curve tests, and the 4-galactosyl-xylose curve are the most used [54, 55].

Genetic Test

This test identifies polymorphisms in the LCT gene through DNA isolation from a blood sample. The identified polymorphisms include LCT13910C > T [59] and LCT-22018G > A [60]. This method does not detect secondary intolerance but is important for distinguishing primary hypolactasia from secondary, to initiate appropriate therapy. Therefore, the genetic test should be performed after confirming lactose intolerance through another method, to exclude or confirm a primary form [51].

Rapid Lactase Test

The rapid lactase test involves biopsies of the post-bulbar duodenal mucosa, which are subsequently incubated with lactose in Petri dishes. Dark blue coloration in the presence of enzymatic activity indicates full activity, light blue indicates partial activity, and no coloration indicates a complete absence of lactase activity, thus indicating severe hypolactasia [51].

Hydrogen Breath Test

Due to its ease of application, the hydrogen breath test is the most accepted method worldwide for assessing LI. The test has a sensitivity of 77.5% and a specificity of 97.6%. It is based on the anaerobic fermentation of lactose by intestinal microbiota in the colon, producing short-chain fatty acids (methane, acetic acid, propionic acid, and butyric acid) and hydrogen. Both methane and hydrogen are absorbed and transported to the lungs via the bloodstream, where they are exhaled and measured [54]. The test involves measuring exhaled hydrogen after fasting and following the ingestion of 25–50 g of lactose, with hydrogen levels measured every 15 min for 3–6 h. An increase in exhaled hydrogen concentration above 20 ppm from baseline suggests hypolactasia [51].

Lactose Tolerance Test

The lactose tolerance test involves an oral challenge followed by blood glucose measurement. Low glucose levels indicate poor digestion, as lactose is not broken down into glucose and galactose; thus, glucose is not detected at high levels in peripheral blood samples [55]. The test involves administering 50 g of lactose to the patient, with subsequent blood glucose measurements before lactose ingestion and at 30-, 60-, and 120-min post-ingestion. This test is rarely performed due to its low sensitivity and specificity. False positive and false negative results occur in 20% of normal subjects [51].

Clinical Management and Therapeutic Options

There are different approaches and therapeutic schemes for managing LI. The first line of management is dietary change, reducing dairy consumption to eliminate the triggering agent without compromising the intake of nutrients, proteins, calcium ions, polyunsaturated fatty acids, and other substances essential for various physiological functions), such as bone remodeling. For congenital lactase deficiency, complete avoidance of lactose is necessary, requiring avoidance of breast milk and lactose-containing formulas. These infants can be given lactose-free formulas using other carbohydrates (e.g., glucose). For patients with other types of lactase deficiency, the goal is to consume between 12 and 15 grams of lactose per day, which is generally well-tolerated.

Another useful option for treating LI is the administration of exogenous lactase, obtained from nonhuman sources (bacterial or fungal). Exogenous lactase, available in capsules, tablets, or emulsions, replaces the native enzyme's functions, improving clinical outcomes in children, adolescents, and adults with LI. One such exogenous lactase is β-galactosidase from the fermentation of *Aspergillus oryzae* [4, 51].

Changes in intestinal flora are another widely used strategy for managing LI. The use of prebiotics has been associated with changes in the relative amounts of colonic microbiota, leading to increased lactose tolerance after treatment with the reintroduction of dairy products. The mechanism associated with prebiotic administration is the development of colonic bacteria that can consume lactose without causing symptoms, possibly due to different metabolic products of the microbiota [55].

Toxic Adverse Reactions to Bovine Milk

Intoxications from consuming cow's milk are not very common. However, since milk is a route for excreting contaminants to which the animal may have been exposed during its upbringing (microorganisms, toxins, antibiotic residues, anti-parasitic agents, hormones, and organophosphate and organochlorine pesticides), the concentration of these contaminants is a critical factor in the incidence of acute or chronic toxicity episodes, depending on the consumption rate of this food. Contamination of milk can occur before milking (indirectly) through pathogens infecting the animal, medications used, or substances present in the feed, or during or after milking (directly) through contamination from the milker's hands or machinery used in milk up to the final industrialization process [61].

Differential Diagnosis

The clinical manifestations of cow's milk allergy (CMA) and lactose intolerance (LI) exhibit significant overlap, often resulting in misdiagnosis. However, CMA can lead to additional symptoms such as skin lesions (e.g., atopic eczema) and respiratory manifestations, which are not observed in LI. Conversely, LI is characterized by the absence of any associated immunological mechanisms and is more prevalent in adults than in children. A detailed comparison of these two conditions is shown in Table 3.2 [50].

Table 3.2 Differences between cow's milk allergy (CMA) and lactose intolerance (LI)

Feature	Cow's milk allergy (CMA)	Lactose intolerance (LI)
Etiology	Immune-mediated reaction to milk proteins	Enzymatic deficiency (lactase) leading to poor lactose digestion
Age of onset	Common in infants and young children	More common in adults
Symptoms	Skin (eczema, hives), respiratory (wheezing, cough)	Gastrointestinal (bloating, diarrhea, gas)
Immune mechanism	Yes, involving IgE antibodies	No immune mechanism involved
Diagnosis	Skin prick tests, specific IgE tests, oral food challenge	Hydrogen breath test, lactose tolerance test, genetic test
Management	Avoidance of cow's milk proteins, use of hydrolyzed formulas	Reduction of lactose intake, use of lactase supplements
Extraintestinal symptoms	Possible (anaphylaxis, atopic eczema)	Rare, mostly limited to the gastrointestinal tract

Conclusions

Adverse food reactions (AFRs) are increasingly prevalent in modern society, with their etiology and underlying pathophysiological mechanisms serving as critical factors influencing prognosis and the severity of clinical manifestations. Among nontoxic AFRs, cow's milk allergy (CMA) and lactose intolerance (LI) are the most common, often resulting in diagnostic confusion due to the similarity in their clinical presentations. Nevertheless, current diagnostic tools are comprehensive and facilitate thorough patient evaluation. Typically, the presence of clinical manifestations in the skin and respiratory tract helps differentiate LI, which primarily presents with gastrointestinal symptoms. The primary management strategy for CMA involves the elimination of milk from the diet or the use of extensively hydrolyzed formulas. In contrast, the management of LI focuses on dietary modifications that reduce dairy consumption while ensuring adequate intake of essential nutrients, proteins, calcium, polyunsaturated fatty acids, and other vital substances.

Glossary

Glossary of Acronyms

AAAAI American Academy of Allergy, Asthma and Immunology
BMA Bovine Milk Allergy
CAS Caseins
CMA Cow's Milk Allergy
CMP Cow's Milk Proteins
CoMiSS Cow's Milk-related Symptom Score
DCs Dendritic Cells
EHF Extensively Hydrolyzed Formulas
IgE Immunoglobulin E
IFN-γ Interferon Gamma
IL-2 Interleukin 2
LI Lactose Intolerance
LPH Lactase-Phlorizin Hydrolase
SGLT-1 Sodium/Glucose Cotransporter 1
TH2 Type 2 Helper T Cells
TGF-β Transforming Growth Factor Beta
Tregs Regulatory T Cells
WPs Whey Proteins
α-La Alpha-Lactalbumin
β-Lg Beta-Lactoglobulin

Glossary of Terms

AAAAI American Academy of Allergy, Asthma and Immunology.

Adverse Food Reactions An abnormal clinical response evidenced in an organism because of ingestion, contact, or inhalation of a food, its derivatives, or one of its additives, which may be perfectly tolerated by the majority of people.

Caseins Insoluble proteins in mammalian milk that have high biological value and a significant amount of phosphate.

Cow's Milk A yellowish-white liquid that has become very important in human nutrition.

Cow's Milk Allergy A disease characterized by an exaggerated immune response to milk proteins, primarily β-lactoglobulin and casein.

Cow's Milk Proteins Biomolecules that include caseins, whey proteins, lactoglobulins, Immunoglobulins A, G, M, Lactoferrin among others.

Cytotoxic T Cells Also known as CD8+ cytotoxic T lymphocytes, these are immune system cells capable of inducing apoptosis in other cells (virus-infected, cancerous) through immunological synapse.

Dendritic Cells Cells that express class I and II MHC antigen-presenting molecules and functionally induce the activation and proliferation of T lymphocytes to which they present antigens.

EAACI European Academy of Allergy and Clinical Immunology.

Extensively Hydrolyzed Formulas Hypoallergenic formulas based on cow's milk with a high degree of protein hydrolysis, the primary treatment option for pediatric patients with Cow's Milk Allergy (CMA), in cases where breastfeeding is not possible or does not show improvement with exclusive breastfeeding and elimination of cow's milk from the mother's diet.

Human Breast Milk A biological fluid that adapts to the nutritional needs of infants according to time and their growth.

Hypersensitivity Reaction Specific immune responses that produce marked clinical conditions in certain individuals (atopics), where the immune system reacts abnormally to noninfectious and harmless substances for most organisms.

Type 1 Helper T Cells Lymphocytes that secrete interferon γ (IFN-γ) and interleukin 2 (IL-2).

Type 2 Helper T Cells Lymphocytes that remain in the lymphoid tissue and assist in the activation of B lymphocytes. They play an important role in hypersensitivity reactions.

Whey Proteins The soluble portion of milk proteins, whose main components are β-lactoglobulin, α-lactalbumin, Glycomacropeptide, Immunoglobulins.

Xenobiotic Any foreign substance in an organism that is not naturally produced by it or is not expected to be present at a particular concentration.

References

1. Caminero A. Reacciones adversas a los alimentos: ¿Cuál es el papel de los microorganismos? Acta Gastroenterol Latinoam. 2021;51(3):259–70.
2. Antolín-Amérigo D, Rodríguez-Rodríguez M, Barbarroja-Escudero J, Sánchez-González MJ. Reacciones alérgicas a alimentos. Med. 2013;11(29):1788–96.
3. Ruiz Sánchez JG, Palma Milla S, Pelegrina Cortés B, López Plaza B, Bermejo López LM, Gómez-Candela C. A global vision of adverse reactions to foods: food allergy and food intolerance. Nutr Hosp. 2018;35(4):102–8.
4. Miles EA. Adverse reactions to cow's milk. Milk and dairy foods. Elsevier Inc.; 2020. p. 271–97.
5. Rua L, Sawsan F, Hamadi A, Mohamed A, Haterm M. Characteristics of cow milk proteins and the effect of processing on their allergenicity. IntchOpen.
6. Caira S, Pizzano R, Picariello G, Pinto G, Cuollo M, Chianese L, et al. Allergenicity of milk proteins. INTECH. 2012:4.
7. Cubides-Munévar ÁM, Linero-Terán AS, Saldarriaga-Vélez MA, Umaña-Bautista EJ, Betancourt EAV. Diagnostic and therapeutic approach to cow's milk protein allergy. Rev Colomb Gastroenterol. 2020;35(1):92–103.
8. Shoormasti RS, Fazlollahi MR, Barzegar S. The most common cow 's milk allergenic proteins with respect to allergic symptoms in Iranian patients. Iran J Allergy Asthma Immunol. 2016;15:161–5.
9. Flom JD, Sicherer SH. Epidemiology of cow's milk allergy. Nutrients. 2019;11:5.
10. Mousan G, Kamat D. Cow's milk protein allergy. Clin Pediatr (Phila). 2016;55(11):1054–63.
11. Halken S, Sicherer SH. Epidemiology of cow's milk allergy gastrointestinal symptoms. Nutrients. 2019;11(1051):2–14.
12. Jo J, Garssen J, Knippels L, Sandalova E. Role of cellular immunity in cow's milk allergy: pathogenesis, tolerance induction, and beyond. Hindawi Publishing Corporation Mediators of Inflammation; 2014.
13. Ashton G. Cow's milk protein allergy. Paediatr Child Health. 2020:1–6.
14. Espa S. Diagnosis and management of cow's milk protein allergy in Turkey: Region-specific recommendations by an expert panel. Allergologia et immunopathologic. 2020;48(2):202–10.
15. Hochwallner H, Schulmeister U, Swoboda I, Spitzauer S, Valenta R. Cow's milk allergy: from allergens to new forms of diagnosis, therapy and prevention. Methods. 2014;66(1):22–33.
16. Villa C, Costa J, Oliveira MBPP, Mafra I. Bovine milk allergens: a comprehensive review. Compr Rev Food Sci Food Saf. 2018;17(1):137–64.
17. Roncada P, Piras C, Soggiu A, Turk R, Urbani A, Bonizzi L. Farm animal milk proteomics. J Proteome. 2012;75(14):4259–74.
18. Pisanu S, Ghisaura S, Pagnozzi D, Biosa G, Tanca A, Roggio T, et al. The sheep milk fat globule membrane proteome. J Proteome. 2011;74(3):350–8.
19. Pereira PC. Milk nutritional composition and its role in human health. Nutrition. 2014;30(6):619–27.
20. Kowalski IM, Zwierzchowski G, Micin J, Pieroz B. Characteristics of cow's milk proteins including allergenic properties and methods for its reduction. Pol Ann Med. 2013;20:69–76.
21. Docena GH, Fernandez R, Chirdo FG, Fossati CA. Identification of casein as the major allergenic and antigenic protein of cow's milk. Allergy Eur J Allergy Clin Immunol. 1996;51(6):412–6.
22. Candreva ÁM, Ferrer-Navarro M, Bronsoms S, Quiroga A, Curciarello R, Cauerhff A, et al. Identification of cross-reactive B-cell epitopes between Bos d 9.0101(Bos Taurus) and Gly m 5.0101 (Glycine max) by epitope mapping MALDI-TOF MS. Proteomics. 2017;17(15–16):15–6.
23. Candreva AM, Smaldini PL, Curciarello R, Cauerhff A, Fossati CA, Docena GH, et al. Cross-reactivity between P34 and bovine caseins AAIR. Allergy Asthma Immunol Res. 2015;7(1):60–8.

24. Candreva ÁM, Ferrer-navarro M, Bronsoms S, Quiroga A, Curciarello R, Cauerhff A, et al. Identification of cross-reactive B-cell epitopes between Bos d 9 0101 (Bos Taurus) and Gly m 5. 0101 (Glycine max) by epitope mapping MALDI-TOF MS. 2017;0101:1–33.
25. Roy D, Ye A, Moughan PJ, Singh H. Composition, structure, and digestive dynamics of milk from different species—a review. Front Nutr. 2020;7:1–17.
26. Fontecha J, Recio I. Pilosof AMR. Funcionalidad de Componentes Lácteos. 2009;407
27. Martinez Corzo M. Caracterización, funcionalidad tecnológica y bioactividad de proteínas lácteas glicosiladas vía reacción de maillard. 2010;1–370.
28. Markoska T, Vasiljevic T, Huppertz T. Unravelling conformational aspects of milk protein structure-contributions from nuclear magnetic resonance studies. Food Secur. 2020;9(8):1–19.
29. Chatchatee P, Järvinen KM, Bardina L, Beyer K, Sampson HA. Identification of IgE- and IgG-binding epitopes on αs1-casein: differences patients with persistent and transient cow's milk allergy. J Allergy Clin Immunol. 2001;107(2):379–83.
30. Cerecedo I, Zamora J, Shreffler WG, Lin J, Bardina L, Dieguez MC, et al. Mapping of the IgE and IgG4 sequential epitopes of milk allergens with a peptide microarray-based immunoassay. J Allergy Clin Immunol. 2008;122(3):589–94.
31. Lisson M, Lochnit G, Erhardt G. Genetic variants of bovine β- and κ-casein result in different immunoglobulin E-binding epitopes after in vitro gastrointestinal digestion. J Dairy Sci. 2013;96(9):5532–43.
32. Chatchatee P, Järvinen KM, Bardina L, Vila L, Beyer K, Sampson HA. Identification of IgE and IgG binding epitopes on β- and κ-casein in cow's milk allergic patients. Clin Exp Allergy. 2001;31(8):1256–62.
33. Qi PX, Onwulata CI. Physical properties, molecular structures, and protein quality of texturized whey protein isolate: effect of extrusion moisture content. J Dairy Sci. 2011;94(5):2231–44.
34. Corrochano AR, Buckin V, Kelly PM, Giblin L. Invited review: whey proteins as antioxidants and promoters of cellular antioxidant pathways. J Dairy Sci. 2018;101:4747–61.
35. Nicolás P, Ferreira ML, Lassalle V. A review of magnetic separation of whey proteins and potential application to whey proteins recovery, isolation, and utilization. J Food Eng. 2019;246:7–15.
36. Candreva ÁM, Smaldini PL, Curciarello R, Fossati CA, Docena GH, Petruccelli S. The major soybean allergen Gly m Bd 28K induces hypersensitivity reactions in mice sensitized to cow's milk proteins. J Agric Food Chem. 2016;64(7):1590–9.
37. Docena GH, Fernandez R, Chirdo FG, Fossati CA. Identification of casein as the major allergenic and antigenic protein of cow's milk. Allergy. 1996;51(6):412–6.
38. Curciarello R, Smaldini PL, Candreva AM, González V, Parisi G, Cauerhff A, et al. Targeting a cross-reactive Gly m 5 soy peptide as responsible for hypersensitivity reactions in a milk allergy mouse model. PLoS One. 2014;9(1):e82341.
39. Sampson HA, O'Mahony L, Burks AW, Plaut M, Lack G, Akdis CA. Mechanisms of food allergy. J Allergy Clin Immunol. 2018;141(1):11–9.
40. Loh W, Tang MLK. The epidemiology of food allergy in the global context. Int J Environ Res Public Health. 2018;15(9)
41. Basu S, Banik BK. Immunology: current research hypersensitivity. An Overview. 2018;October
42. Uzzaman A, Cho SH. Classification of hypersensitivity reactions. 2016;33(3):96–9.
43. Yu W, Freeland DMH, Nadeau KC. Food allergy: immune mechanisms, diagnosis, and immunotherapy. Nat Rev Immunol. 2016;16(12):751–65.
44. Article O. Pooled analysis of the cow's milk-related-symptom-score (CoMiSS). Pediatr Gastroenterol Hepatol Nutr. 2017;20(1):22–6.
45. Vandenplas Y, Mukherjee R, Dupont C, Eigenmann P, Høst A, Kuitunen M, et al. Protocol for the validation of sensitivity and specificity of the cow's Milk-related symptom score (CoMiSS) against open food challenge in a single-blinded, prospective, multicentre trial in infants. BMJ Open. 2018;8(5):e019968.

46. Vandenplas Y, Belohlavkova S, Enninger A, Frühauf P, Makwana N, Järvi A. How are infants suspected to have cow milk allergy managed? A real-world study report. Nutrients. 2021;13(9):1–12.
47. Koletzko S, Niggemann B, Arato A, Dias JA, Heuschkel R, Husby S, et al. Diagnostic approach and management of cow's-milk protein allergy in infants and children: Espghan gi committee practical guidelines. J Pediatr Gastroenterol Nutr. 2012;55(2):221–9.
48. Matthai J, Sathiasekharan M, Poddar U, Sibal A, Srivastava A, Waikar Y, et al. Guidelines on diagnosis and management of cow's milk protein allergy. Indian Pediatr. 2020;7:723.
49. D'auria E, Salvatore S, Acunzo M, Peroni D, Pendezza E, Di Profio E, et al. Hydrolyzed formulas in the management of cow's milk allergy: new insights, pitfalls, and tips. Nutrients. 2021;13(8):1–21.
50. Rangel AHDN, Sales DC, Urbano SA, Galvão JGB, de Andrade Neto JC, de Macêdo CS. Lactose intolerance and cow's milk protein allergy. Food Sci Technol. 2016;36(2):179–87.
51. Catanzaro R, Sciuto M, Marotta F. Lactose intolerance: an update on its pathogenesis, diagnosis, and treatment. Nutr Res. 2021;89:23–34.
52. Heine RG, Alrefaee F, Bachina P, De Leon JC, Geng L, Gong S, et al. Lactose intolerance and gastrointestinal cow's milk allergy in infants and children—common misconceptions revisited. World Allergy Organ J. 2017;10(1):1–8.
53. Brown-Esters O, Mc Namara P, Savaiano D. Dietary and biological factors influencing lactose intolerance. Int Dairy J [Internet]. 2012;22(2):98–103.
54. Martínez Vázquez SE, Nogueira de Rojas JR, Remes Troche JM, Coss Adame E, Rivas Ruíz R, Uscanga Domínguez LF. The importance of lactose intolerance in individuals with gastrointestinal symptoms. Rev Gastroenterol México (English Ed). 2020;85(3):321–31.
55. Jansson-Knodell CL, Krajicek EJ, Savaiano DA, Shin AS. Lactose intolerance: a concise review to skim the surface. Mayo Clin Proc [Internet]. 2020;95(7):1499–505.
56. Hertzler S, Savaiano DA, Dilk A, Jackson KA, Bhriain SN, Suarez FL. Nutrient considerations in lactose intolerance [internet]. In: Fourth Edi. Nutrition in the prevention and treatment of disease. Elsevier Inc.; 2017. p. 875–92.
57. Szilagyi A, Walker C, Thomas MG. Lactose intolerance and other related food sensitivities. lactose: evolutionary role, health effects, and applications. Elsevier Inc.; 2019. p. 113–53.
58. Wanes D, Husein DM, Naim HY. Congenital lactase deficiency: mutations, functional and biochemical implications, and future perspectives. Nutrients. 2019;11(2):1–9.
59. Alharbi O, El-Sohemy A. Lactose intolerance (LCT-13910C > T) genotype is associated with plasma 25-hydroxyvitamin D concentrations in Caucasians: a Mendelian randomization study. J Nutr. 2017;147(6):1063–9.
60. Raz M, Sharon Y, Yerushalmi B, Birk R. Frequency of LCT-13910C/T and LCT-22018G/A single nucleotide polymorphisms associated with adult-type hypolactasia/lactase persistence among Israelis of different ethnic groups. Gene. 2013;519(1):67–70.
61. Lopes JRG, Riet-Correa F, Medeiros RMT. Phytotoxins eliminated by milk: a review. Pasquil Vet Bras. 2019;39(4):231–7.

Chapter 4
Intolerance, Allergies, and Acute Intoxication to Alcoholic Beverages

José Dussan Ordoñez

Introduction

An alcoholic beverage is any liquid suitable for human consumption that contains ethanol derived from the fermentation of sugars [1]. Additionally, it contains other organic and inorganic components derived from the type of raw materials used in fermentation and the industrial or artisanal distillation processes to obtain the final product: beer, wine, whiskey, aguardiente, rum, etc. [2]. It has no nutritional value due to the minimal or absent contribution of macro or micronutrients [3], but it does have a high caloric content quantified at seven kilocalories per gram of alcohol (see formula) [4], and its consumption is primarily for recreational purposes. In Colombia, the legislation refers to two additional aspects: an ethanol level above 2.5 alcoholometric degrees and no therapeutic indication to be considered a beverage, classifying it as an alcoholic beverage [5]. The World Health Organization (WHO), in its 2018 report on the global status of alcohol and health, estimated that more than two billion people worldwide consume alcoholic beverages, while the total per capita ethanol consumption in people over 15 years old increased from 5.5 liters in 2005 to 6.4 liters in 2016. By 2025, it is projected that consumption will rise to 7 liters per person [6]. In the 2013 national survey on psychoactive substance use in Colombia, it was found that 87% of the surveyed population had consumed an alcoholic beverage at least once [7]. This indicates many people exposed to ethanol and other substances contained in these beverages, increasing the number of adverse reactions that compromise the health of consumers.

J. D. Ordoñez (✉)
Faculty of Health, Universidad del Sinú, Cartagena, Colombia
e-mail: Jose.dussan@Unisinu.edu.co

M. G. Múnera Gómez et al. (eds.), *Allergies, Poisoning and Intolerance to Common Substances*, https://doi.org/10.1007/978-3-031-93658-6_4

Historical Review

There is evidence of the consumption of alcoholic beverages dating back 10,000 years, primarily in Western cultures near the Mediterranean. Mead was perhaps the first alcoholic beverage, resulting from the accidental mixing of collected fruits with water, with fermentation occurring during storage. This phenomenon was attributed to the gods and became the everyday "spiritual food" for communication with the supreme beings of the universe. In Egyptian and Greco-Roman civilizations, wine and beer were present at all kinds of ceremonies and gatherings and were even used as treatments for some diseases. For example, in Egypt, the most common beverage was beer, which, besides being consumed, was used for various everyday purposes such as weaning infants, as an initiation rite for teenagers, and washing the dead before embalming them [8]. The excessive consumption of alcoholic beverages was documented in ancient times; Hippocrates made the first description of alcohol intoxication and the behavioral changes in a person with alcoholism. In pre-Islamic Arabia, wine was consumed with poetry or before and after a battle [9]. Distillation was known to the Greeks and Romans, but the Arabs perfected the technique, building more advanced stills that produced beverages with higher alcohol content. The first European descriptions of distilled alcohol date from around 1100. The word "alcohol" comes from the Arabic "al-Kohol," meaning "fine powder" [10], referring to any element refined to its essence. The first distillation produced a beverage with 60% alcohol by volume, called "aqua ardens" (firewater); a second distillation increased the concentration to 96%, and the final product was known as "aqua vitae," or water of life. Initially, this distilled alcohol was mixed with herbs to be sold as medicine, and during the Black Death that devastated the European population between 1348 and 1352, the habit of consuming these higher concentration beverages spread, whereas the custom had previously been to consume wine and beer [11]. From the fifteenth century to the present day, fermented and distilled beverages have been socioculturally linked to celebrations [12] but also to social violence and the general deterioration of consumers' health.

Types of Alcoholic Beverages

Alcoholic beverages can be classified into fermented and distilled. Fermented beverages include wine, beer, and cider, which are produced by the glycolysis of sugars from fruits and grains. The ethanol concentration in fermented beverages does not exceed 15 alcoholometric degrees. Distilled beverages include aguardiente, rum, vodka, whiskey, gin, tequila, etc. These are obtained by separating the different components of previously fermented products through heat. They exceed 15 degrees of alcohol by volume and can reach concentrations between 30 and 50 alcoholometric degrees [13, 14].

Ethanol

Ethanol, or ethyl alcohol, is a colorless, water-soluble liquid that easily crosses the plasma membrane and is the main component of alcoholic beverages, with its concentration varying depending on the type of beverage [15]. After ingestion, ethanol is well absorbed in the gastrointestinal tract, with one-fifth of the dose absorbed in the stomach and the rest absorbed in the small intestine. Within 60 min, up to 90% of the ethanol is already in the bloodstream [16]. Several factors can modify the absorption rate, such as the presence of food, gastric emptying motility, the concentration of ethanol, and the calories of the beverage. For example, beer and wine are absorbed more slowly on an empty stomach than whiskey or vodka. Therefore, blood ethanol peaks after ingestion are variable and also depend on the type of alcoholic beverage [17]. Ethyl alcohol has a body distribution volume similar to the amount of water in the body, between 0.6 L and 0.7 L/kg, depending on lean body weight and the degree of hydration of the person. In women, the distribution volume is smaller due to the higher amount of adipose tissue [18]. Alcohol metabolism primarily occurs through the oxidative pathway in hepatocytes with the action of the cytosolic enzyme Alcohol Dehydrogenase (ADH), which is also expressed in other tissues such as the stomach and brain [19]. Other oxidative pathway routes intervene to a lesser extent, including cytochrome p450 isoform CYP2E1 and catalases. The product of these oxidative reactions is acetaldehyde, which is then metabolized by the mitochondrial enzyme Aldehyde Dehydrogenase (ALDH) to form acetate [20]. Acetate is a precursor of acetyl CoA, which enters the Krebs cycle.

Ethanol Elimination

Ethanol is primarily eliminated by the liver, but it can also be excreted through urine, sweat, and in the exhaled air from the lungs. Initially, the alcohol dehydrogenase enzyme complex in hepatocytes quickly becomes saturated, and the elimination rate will be constant and independent of ethanol concentration (zero-order kinetics). When ethanol concentration is lower, the enzyme system is not saturated, and the elimination rate remains unchanged, maintaining the metabolic rate of ethanol (first-order kinetics). On average, a person can eliminate 0.10–0.25 g/l/h [21], but there are differences between social drinkers and alcoholics, with the latter having a higher elimination rate. Other factors that modify the elimination rate include ADH polymorphism, niacin deficiency, advanced liver diseases, body temperature, and certain medications [22].

Ethanol's Effects on the Nervous System

When ethanol reaches the nervous system, it disrupts the balance between the inhibitory action of GABAergic pathways and the excitatory action of glutamatergic pathways. Acute exposure decreases the sensitivity of GABA receptors and suppresses glutamate receptors. Ethanol also binds to GABA receptors, triggering inhibitory functions, manifested as sedation, cognitive dysfunction, and decreased coordination [23]. The initial stimulating effects during alcohol consumption are due to dopamine action on the prefrontal cortex and the neuronal reward system. Serotonin and the endocannabinoid system are also altered during acute ethanol consumption [24]. Chronic consumption alters histone acetylation in limbic areas and can contribute to alcohol use disorder, fragmenting REM sleep and causing short and poor-quality sleep [25].

Ethanol and Gut Health

Ethanol causes dysbiosis, damaging the intestinal microbiota. These bacteria start generating endotoxins/lipopolysaccharides that cause inflammation of the small and large intestine mucosa. This inflammatory process activates apoptosis of epithelial mucosal cells, leading to the loss of microvilli and ulcerations. The inflammatory process ultimately affects the immune response of the intestinal tissue, increasing the possibility of extraintestinal endotoxin circulation [26]. Intestinal mucosal permeability processes are related to lesions on tight and adherens junctions of the intestinal epithelium. Oxidation of tubulin, damage to the microtubule cytoskeleton, activation of nitric oxide synthase enzyme, and NF-κB signaling (nuclear factor kappa-light-chain-enhancer of activated B cells) are activated by acetaldehyde, disrupting the intestinal barrier and increasing the risk of hepatic colonization by enteric bacteria [27]. Acute ethanol ingestion is associated with elevated proinflammatory cytokines such as interleukin-1 β (IL-1β), interleukin-6 (IL-6), tumor necrosis factor-α (TNF-α), and the activation of Toll-Like Receptors 3 and 4, implicating the innate immunity response [28]. Another impact on the immune system is the altered phagocytosis of alveolar macrophages, becoming a risk factor for pneumonia [29]. The complement system is also activated at the hepatic level by ethanol exposure, contributing to inflammation [27].

Mitochondrial Effects and Oxidative Stress

In hepatocytes, mitochondrial levels of nicotinamide adenine dinucleotide (NAD+), a coenzyme necessary for cellular energy metabolism, decrease due to ethanol metabolism-induced oxidative stress, increasing the conversion of NAD+ to NADH (the reduced form by electron gain). This impairs mitochondrial homeostasis [30] and

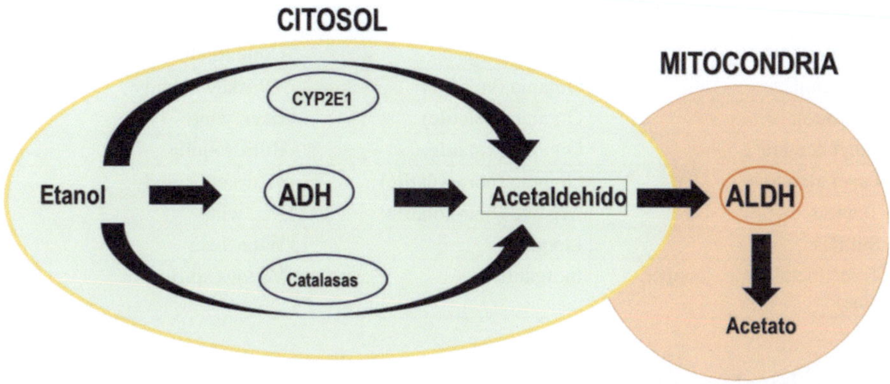

Fig. 4.1 The figure illustrates ethanol metabolism in the cytosol and mitochondria. In the cytosol, ethanol is converted into acetaldehyde mainly by the enzyme alcohol dehydrogenase (ADH), with catalases and CYP2E1 also playing a role. Acetaldehyde then enters the mitochondria, where it is transformed into acetate by the enzyme aldehyde dehydrogenase (ALDH). The resulting acetate is less toxic and can be used by the body to produce energy

increases the production of reactive oxygen species (ROS). Carnitine's function of transporting long-chain fatty acids to the mitochondria for β-oxidation is also affected, increasing lipid peroxidation and further disrupting energy metabolism [31]. Glutathione, acting as a hepatic antioxidant, is depleted due to the mitochondrial toxicity of ethanol and its metabolites, leaving hepatocytes vulnerable to deleterious damage by sensitization to TNF-α and inducing cell death [32]. Additionally, the expression of genes promoting fat accumulation, such as Sterol Regulatory Element-Binding Protein 1 (SREBF1), increases, while the inhibition of other genes involved in fat metabolism, like Peroxisome Proliferator-Activated Receptor-α (PPAR-α), occurs. This fat infiltration in liver tissue leads to organ dysfunction [33] (Fig. 4.1).

Intolerance and Allergies to Alcoholic Beverages

In the composition of alcoholic beverages, in addition to ethanol, we can find various organic substances (volatile and non-volatile) and some inorganic components (trace elements) capable of interacting with several metabolic pathways in our bodies. These substances are called congeners (see Table 4.1) [34, 35]. Generally, darker beverages such as aged rum, red wine, and whiskey have a higher concentration of congeners than lighter-colored beverages. For example, bourbon has 37 times more congeners than vodka. These differences in the non-ethanol components of beverages have clinical importance in the severity of hangovers [36]. People report that consuming certain alcoholic beverages causes headaches, dry mouth, nausea, and general physical discomfort, but these hangover symptoms do not occur when they consume other types of beverages with the same ethanol percentage.

Table 4.1 Non-ethanol components of alcoholic beverages

Components	Type	Common beverages
Methanol	Organic (volatile)	Whiskey, brandy
Acetone	Organic (volatile)	Beer, wine
Ethyl acetate	Organic (volatile)	Rum, tequila
Fusel alcohols	Organic (non-volatile)	Whiskey, brandy
Tannins	Organic (non-volatile)	Red wine
Sulfites	Inorganic	Wine, beer
Trace metals (e.g., copper, zinc)	Inorganic	Various spirits

Acute Intolerance to Alcoholic Beverages

Acute intolerance to alcoholic beverages is directly related to the accumulation of acetaldehyde in the body, either due to excessive intake (beverages with high concentrations of congeners such as histamine, sulfites, tyramine) [37] or decreased ALDH activity (people carrying the ALDH2 genotype). Acetaldehyde is considered a cytotoxic molecule that promotes the release of pro-inflammatory cytokines and can bind to certain proteins (adducts) [38] and damage DNA, generating mutations [39]. The body's reaction to the increased presence of this ethanol metabolite in tissues involves the release of substances such as epinephrine, norepinephrine, histamine, and bradykinin. The patient experiences nausea, dizziness, dyspnea, tachycardia, increased blood pressure, and peripheral vasodilation, which manifests as facial flushing and a sensation of heat. Disulfiram is a drug that inhibits the enzyme aldehyde dehydrogenase and is used as a treatment for people with alcohol use disorders, causing the unpleasant clinical manifestations mentioned above [40] (Fig. 4.2).

The figure shows ethanol metabolism and the effect of disulfiram. Ethanol is converted into acetaldehyde by alcohol dehydrogenase (ADH). Acetaldehyde is then transformed into acetate by aldehyde dehydrogenase 2 (ALDH2). Disulfiram inhibits ALDH2, leading to an accumulation of acetaldehyde, which causes unpleasant effects when alcohol is consumed.

Another type of adverse effect associated with alcoholic beverages is hypersensitivity reactions, which can be triggered by any component of the drink that has previously sensitized our immune system. The frequency of these reactions is increasing among social drinkers due to the use of different ingredients added to beverages during their manufacturing process (clarifying agents such as casein, preservatives like potassium metabisulfite, etc.) to achieve special characteristics in flavor, aroma, body, and color. Frequent consumers of alcoholic beverages have been found to have elevated levels of immunoglobulin E (IgE) and interleukin 8 (IL-8), leading to a baseline state of sensitization in the body and a higher frequency of airway hyperreactivity episodes [41]. In people diagnosed with rosacea, these beverages can exacerbate the dermatological condition after consumption. Studies have shown that ethanol is directly related to the induction of mast cell

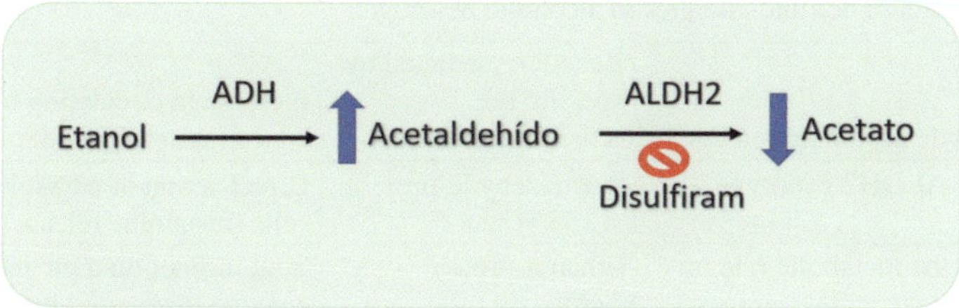

Fig. 4.2 Altered acetaldehyde metabolism and its accumulation

degranulation, raising histamine levels, inhibiting the enzyme diamine oxidase that metabolizes histamine, activating prostaglandin receptors, and the opioid system releasing endogenous opioids. All these interactions cause alcohol-induced urticaria and pseudo-allergic manifestations due to increased plasma histamine. Biopsies from patients with alcohol-induced dermatitis have found mast cells, polymorphonuclear cells, and eosinophils, typical findings of type IV hypersensitivity reactions.

Allergies with elevated specific IgE are more frequently related to congeners and acetaldehyde; this metabolite can form acetaldehyde-protein complexes that act as haptens, triggering an immune response. There are reported cases of anaphylaxis to alcoholic beverages confirmed by elevated tryptase levels, although these severe clinical conditions remain rare. Double-blind, placebo-controlled clinical trials of ethanol hypersensitivity showed that "allergic" reactions appeared at cumulative doses of ethanol, suggesting mechanisms not associated with IgE [42]. Type I hypersensitivity reactions have been reported in association with barley malt protein [43], nonspecific lipid transfer proteins [44], plant additives such as cilantro [45], yeast Saccharomyces cerevisiae [46], grape glycoproteins [47], contamination of beverages by hymenopteran insect proteins [48], thaumatin-like proteins, and endokinase 4A [42].

Identification and Differentiation of Adverse Reactions to Alcoholic Beverages

To identify and differentiate adverse reactions to alcoholic beverages in patients (see Table 4.2), it is essential to document the type of beverage (fermented or distilled), the quantity consumed, and the time elapsed since the last intake. Additionally, it is important to know if there is any underlying disease or history of food allergies, if the patient is taking medications, and what type of beverage they usually consume. If a person has a history of tolerance to different beverages, for example, they have previously consumed beer and vodka, it is possible that the current clinical picture of intolerance or allergy is not due to ethanol and its metabolites but rather to some congener of the newly consumed beverage. It should be noted that habitual drinkers may develop haptenization processes with ethanol and congeners, facilitated by medications, diseases, or other substances. These individuals may have been drinking for a long time and, due to some new condition, start developing

Table 4.2 Intolerance and allergies to alcoholic beverages

Acetaldehyde accumulation due to:	Reaction mediated by specific IgE sensitization to:	Increase in circulating histamine concentration secondary to:
Possessing ALDH2 genotype	Acetaldehyde-protein	Direct action of ethanol on mast cells (histamine release)
Exceeding the metabolic rate by excessive intake and beverages with high acetaldehyde content	Ethanol-protein (very rare)	Inhibition of diamine oxidase enzyme (decreased histamine metabolism)
Pharmacological inhibition of ALDH (disulfiram) [54]	Lipid transfer protein (most common allergen)	Beverages with high biogenic amine content
Drug interaction: Metronidazole, nitrofurantoin, trimethoprim + sulfamethoxazole among others.	Glycoproteins, proteins, and vegetable-origin additives	
	Contaminant proteins	
Most frequent clinical manifestations are:	Most frequent clinical manifestations are:	Most frequent clinical manifestations are:
Headache, dizziness	Anaphylaxis [55]	Headache
Nausea, vomiting	Angioedema, itching, redness, hives	Nausea, vomiting
Dyspnea, wheezing	Bronchial hyperreactivity, stridor	Abdominal pain
Chest pain, tachycardia, increased blood pressure, sensation of increased body temperature with facial flushing	Cardiovascular shock, peripheral hypoperfusion	Erythema, itching, dermatitis, hives
General malaise	Hypoxemia/cyanosis	Dyspnea, rhinorrhea, asthma attack
Severe clinical cases may present with ataxia, altered consciousness, and seizures		Conjunctival hyperemia
		High plasma histamine concentrations can lead to tachycardia, ventricular arrhythmias, laryngeal edema, and severe hypotension

allergies. Adverse reactions to alcoholic beverages have different molecular mechanisms, reflecting the clinical variability observed in patients after consumption.

Acute Alcohol Intoxication

Ethanol is the most widely consumed socially accepted psychoactive substance in the world. It has a wide age range among consumers, and excessive intake is linked to a higher incidence of traffic accidents, various forms of violence, the risk of using

Table 4.3 Neurological alterations according to blood ethanol level

Ethanol blood level	Clinical manifestations
50–100 mg/dl	Euphoria, loquacity, difficulty concentrating, and decreased judgment capacity
100–150 mg/dl	Difficulty maintaining balance, nystagmus, diplopia, dysarthria, and ataxia
150–300 mg/dl	Lethargy, stupor, clouding of consciousness, incoherent speech, and vomiting
300–400 mg/dl	Coma, respiratory depression, hypotension, hypothermia, and hypoglycemia

other illicit drugs, disability during productive life years, and increased overall mortality. Acute intoxication occurs when the amount of ethyl alcohol consumed exceeds the liver's elimination capacity, causing levels of blood alcohol and its metabolites that alter the nervous system, including the mental sphere. To approximate the amount of alcohol ingested by a patient with alcohol intoxication, the concept of a standard drink (units) containing 12–14 grams of ethanol is used. This corresponds to about 340 ml of beer at 5%, 150 ml of wine at 10%, or 45 ml of distilled spirits at 40% [49]. To reach a blood ethanol level of 60 mg/dl, three standard drinks need to be consumed within an hour. At this level of blood alcohol concentration, individuals initially experience disinhibition, increased sociability and confidence, slight alteration in attention, and may have episodes of euphoria. There is no international definition specifying the volume at which acute intoxication is considered, but behavioral changes due to inhibitory action on the cerebral cortex can indicate toxicity as blood ethanol levels increase (see Table 4.3) [50]. Acute alterations in patients who consume ethyl beverages depend on the volume ingested, absorption capacity, metabolism, and elimination [51]. The diagnosis of intoxication is made with the clinical history and physical examination showing the involvement of central nervous system functions. The DSM-V uses four guiding pillars for the clinical diagnosis of acute intoxication: (1) recent alcohol intake; (2) clinically significant problematic behavior or psychological changes during or after alcohol consumption; (3) signs of intoxication including slurred speech, lack of coordination, unsteady gait, nystagmus, conjunctival injection, impaired attention or memory, stupor, or coma; (4) the signs and symptoms are not attributable to another medical condition and are not better explained by another mental disorder, including intoxication with another substance [52]. Anterograde amnesia is a common feature of the intoxicated patient, due to the dysfunction in the consolidation process of memory in areas of the hippocampus in the temporal lobe under the influence of ethanol. Other consequences include sensory-perceptual alterations, difficulty in fluent communication, dysregulation of operational capacity for work and executive functions. It has been shown that alcohol consumption shortens sleep phases and exacerbates sleep apnea during intoxicated states and with excessive chronic alcohol consumption [53]. Ethanol also causes irritation or injury to the gastrointestinal mucosa, manifested clinically by esophagitis, gastritis, gastric ulcers, even hematemesis due to a longitudinal tear in the mucosa at the gastroesophageal junction (Mallory-Weiss syndrome) [56], or a rupture of the esophagus (Boerhaave syndrome). Patients with repeated and excessive consumption of alcoholic beverages, along with high-fat foods, develop a risk factor for acute pancreatitis and alcoholic hepatitis. Long-term consumption can lead to hepatic steatosis (fatty liver), liver cirrhosis, and cancer [57]. Although low-dose ethanol consumption is considered cardioprotective, studies indicate the risk of cardiotoxicity in the medium to long term if consumption exceeds 30 grams per day. These elevated levels are associated with increased blood pressure, cardiac arrhythmias, and structural heart damage [51].

Alcohol also causes metabolic acidosis due to the elevation of keto acids and lactic acid and interferes with both the decrease in electrolyte absorption and the increase in their urinary excretion, leading to hyponatremia, hypokalemia, hypocalcemia, hypophosphatemia, and hypomagnesemia as recorded in blood tests [58]. It also inhibits gluconeogenesis enzymes due to excess NADH and increases blood flow in the pancreatic microcirculation, releasing more insulin. These two events together cause hypoglycemia in intoxicated patients, with a risk of seizures [16, 59]. Dehydration is a constant in intoxicated patients, but intravenous rehydration must be done cautiously because cases of pontine myelinolysis (damage to the oligodendrocytes of the brainstem pons) have been reported secondary to fluid replacement with isotonic crystalloids for stabilizing intoxicated patients with normonatremia [60].

Acute ethanol intoxication has a multisystemic impact on the individual's health and can have fatal consequences if the diagnosis is not made promptly or if the value of the clinical signs and symptoms indicating the severity of the condition is underestimated. A recommendation made by the Guide for the Management of Toxicological Emergencies from the Ministry of Health in Colombia is that patients intoxicated by alcohol should be observed for at least 6 h in the medical facility [16]. The clinical approach to these patients should consider an effective comprehensive management plan that reduces the likelihood of a recurring intoxication event.

The consumption of alcoholic beverages is a topic of medical and legal importance. New products are continually being developed based on mixtures of raw or processed materials to cater to a wide variety of tastes and preferences. Many consumers of these beverages lack sufficient information about the products they are consuming. Labels on alcoholic beverages do not report the calories per volume consumed, the presence and quantity of congeners, and the additional ingredients used during the manufacturing process. This can complicate the process of making an appropriate diagnosis and managing adverse reactions following consumption. The continuous and excessive exposure of our bodies to this wide range of chemical substances, which have the potential to interact with many metabolic pathways, sensitize our immune system, decrease nutrient absorption, increase electrolyte elimination, and generate toxic metabolites, creates an academic need for healthcare personnel to stay updated on the toxicological information of these xenobiotics. Considering innovations in fermented and distilled beverages is essential to provide necessary and timely care to patients who present to emergency services with clinical symptoms of intolerance, allergies, or intoxication due to alcoholic beverages.

Glossary

Glossary of Acronyms

AAAAI American Academy of Allergy, Asthma and Immunology
ADH Alcohol Dehydrogenase
ALDH Aldehyde Dehydrogenase
CMA Cow's Milk Allergy
CMP Cow's Milk Proteins
CoMiSS Cow's Milk-related Symptom Score
DSM-V Diagnostic and Statistical Manual of Mental Disorders, Fifth Edition
EAACI European Academy of Allergy and Clinical Immunology
EHF Extensively Hydrolyzed Formulas
GABA Gamma-Aminobutyric Acid
IgE Immunoglobulin E
LI Lactose Intolerance
LPH Lactase-Phlorizin Hydrolase
NAD Nicotinamide Adenine Dinucleotide
NAD+ Non-reduced Nicotinamide Adenine Dinucleotide
NADH Reduced Nicotinamide Adenine Dinucleotide
REM Rapid Eye Movement (Sleep)
SGLT-1 Sodium/glucose Cotransporter 1
TH2 Type 2 Helper T cells
TNF-α Tumor Necrosis Factor alpha

Glossary of Terms

ADH Alcohol dehydrogenase, a zinc-containing enzyme that oxidizes primary and secondary alcohols in the cytosol of cells in the presence of non-reduced nicotinamide adenine dinucleotide (NAD+). ADH converts ethyl alcohol to acetaldehyde.

ALDH Aldehyde dehydrogenase, a mitochondrial enzyme that oxidizes an aldehyde in the presence of non-reduced nicotinamide adenine dinucleotide (NAD+) to an acid (acetate/acetic acid) and reduced nicotinamide adenine dinucleotide (NADH).

Cytochrome p450 A family of microsomal enzymes in the liver involved in the oxidative pathway with two main functions: biosynthesis of steroids, fatty acids, and bile acids, and the metabolism of endogenous substrates and a wide variety of exogenous substances such as toxins and drugs.

Congeners of Alcoholic Beverages Non-ethyl chemical products formed during the fermentation and aging process.

CYP2E1 Isoform of the p450 family of microsomal enzymes.

DSM-V *Diagnostic and Statistical Manual of Mental Disorders* published by the American Psychiatric Association.

GABA Gamma-aminobutyric acid, the main inhibitory neurotransmitter in the brain and spinal cord. It hyperpolarizes the cell and inhibits the transmission of an action potential.

Glutathione A tripeptide with many functions in cells. It conjugates with drugs to make them more soluble for excretion, acts as a cofactor for some enzymes, participates in the rearrangement of protein disulfide bonds, and reduces peroxides.

Alcoholic Strength by Volume The percentage of ethyl alcohol by volume at 20 degrees Celsius.

NAD Nicotinamide adenine dinucleotide. It has the ability to transport electrons and exists in two forms: non-reduced (positive charge) and reduced (negative charge due to gain of an electron).

NAD+ The non-reduced form of nicotinamide adenine dinucleotide.

NADH The reduced form of nicotinamide adenine dinucleotide.

Rosacea An inflammatory dermatological disorder characterized by redness of the skin accompanied by small papule-like lesions, most common on the facial skin.

REM Sleep A stage of sleep characterized by rapid eye movement (REM). It is generally associated with dreaming and the process of memory consolidation.

Tubulin Protein subunit of microtubules.

Volume of Distribution The ratio between the amount of a substance in the body tissues and its concentration in the blood.

References

1. Zhou Y, Zheng J, Li S, Zhou T, Zhang P, Li H, bin. Alcoholic beverage consumption and chronic diseases. Int J Environ Res Public Health. MDPI. 2016;13
2. IARC Working Group on the Evaluation of Carcinogenic Risks to Humans., International Agency for Research on Cancer., National Cancer Institute (U.S.). Alcohol drinking. World Health Organization, International Agency for Research on Cancer; 1988. 416 p.
3. McClain CJ, Rios CD, Condon S, Marsano LS. Malnutrition and alcohol-associated hepatitis. In: Clinics in liver disease, vol. 25. W.B. Saunders; 2021. p. 557–70.
4. de cote Orozco Julia. Las bebidas alcohólicas en la historia de la humanidad. medigraphic [Internet]. 2010 Feb 10 [cited 2022 Jul 30]; Available from: www.medigraphic.org.mx
5. Ministerio de salud y protección social. Decreto No162 de 2021.
6. World Health Organization. Global status report on alcohol and health 2018.
7. de la Espriella Guerrero RA, Rodriguez V, Rincón CJ, Morales DC, Rodríguez SJP, Gómez-Restrepo C. Consumo de alcohol en la población colombiana. Encuesta Nacional de Salud Mental 2015. Rev Colomb Psiquiatr. 2016;45:76–88.
8. Pascual F. Aspectos antropológicos del consumo de bebidas alcohólicas en las culturas mediterráneas [Internet]. 2007. Available from: http://www.redalyc.org/articulo.oa?id=83970203
9. Ayman M Hamdan-Mansour. Alcohol history [Internet]. 2016. Available from: https://www.researchgate.net/publication/310589270

10. Hamdan-Mansour AM. Alcohol history investigating physical, psychological and social Well-being of older persons in Jordan view project knowledge and attitudes of Saudi nurses toward pain management. Strengths and Weaknesses View project. 2016; Available from: https://www.researchgate.net/publication/310589270
11. Valiente-Barderas A. Historia de la destilación. Revista de Educación Química. 1996;
12. Valenzuela Zapata AG, Regalado Pinedo A, Mizoguchi M. Influencia asiática en la producción de mezcal en la costa de Jalisco. El caso de la raicilla. México y la Cuenca del Pacífico [Internet]. 2008;33:91–116. Available from: http://www.mexicoylacuencadelpacifico.cucsh.udg.mx/index.php/mc/article/view/317
13. Simunovic Estay Y. Manual de bebidas alcoholicas y vinagres coleccion de manuales juridicos 1999.
14. Victor Z. Clasificación de bebidas alcohólicas destiladas por absorciometría molecular UV-visible. Santa Rosa, La Pampa: Universidad Nacional de la Pampa; 2012.
15. Velasco Martín Académico de Número A. Farmacología Y toxicología del alcohol etílico, o etanol. Pharmacology and toxicology of ethyl alcohol or ethanol. 2014;
16. Minsalud. Guía para el manejo de emergencias toxicológicas. 2017.
17. Mitchell MC, Teigen EL, Ramchandani VA. Absorption and peak blood alcohol concentration after drinking beer, wine, or spirits. Alcohol Clin Exp Res. 2014;38(5):1200–4.
18. Perry PJ, Doroudgar S, van Dyke P. Ethanol forensic toxicology, vol. 45. J Am Acad Psychiatry Law; 2017.
19. Edenberg HJ, McClintick JN. Alcohol dehydrogenases, aldehyde dehydrogenases, and alcohol use disorders: a critical review, vol. 42. Alcoholism: Clinical and Experimental Research. Blackwell Publishing Ltd; 2018. p. 2281–97.
20. le Daré B, Lagente V, Gicquel T. Ethanol and its metabolites: update on toxicity, benefits, and focus on immunomodulatory effects, vol. 51. Drug Metabolism Reviews. Taylor and Francis Ltd; 2019. p. 545–61.
21. Wunder C, Weber C, Paulke A, Koelzer SC, Holz F, Toennes SW. Endogenous formation of 1-propanol and methanol after consumption of alcoholic beverages. Forensic Sci Int. 2021;1:325.
22. Cederbaum AI. Alcohol metabolism, vol. 16. Clinics in Liver Disease; 2012. p. 667–85.
23. LaHood AJ, Kok SJ. Ethanol toxicity. 2022 Mar 18 [cited 2022 Sep 15]; Available from: https://www.ncbi.nlm.nih.gov/books/NBK557381/
24. Palmer E, Tyacke R, Sastre M, Lingford-Hughes A, Nutt D, Ward RJ. Alcohol hangover: underlying biochemical, inflammatory and neurochemical mechanisms, vol. 54. Alcohol and Alcoholism. Oxford University Press; 2019. p. 196–203.
25. Sharma R, Sahota P, Thakkar MM, Truman Memorial HS. Chronic alcohol exposure reduces acetylated histones in the sleep-wake regulatory brain regions to cause insomnia during withdrawa. Neuropharmacology. 2020;180:108332.
26. Bishehsari F, Magno E, Swanson G, Desai V, Voigt RM, Forsyth CB, et al. Alcohol and gut-derived inflammation. 2017.
27. Gao B, Ahmad MF, Nagy LE. Tsukamoto H. Inflammatory pathways in alcoholic steatohepatitis.
28. Lawrimore CJ, Crews FT. Ethanol, TLR3, and TLR4 agonists have unique innate immune responses in neuron-like SH-SY5Y and microglia-like BV2. Alcohol Clin Exp Res. 2017;41(5):939–54.
29. Kaphalia L, Srinivasan MP, Kakumanu RD, Kaphalia BS, Calhoun WJ. Ethanol exposure impairs AMPK signaling and phagocytosis in human alveolar macrophages: role of ethanol metabolism. Alcohol Clin Exp Res. 2019;43(8):1682–94.
30. Wang S, Wan T, Ye M, Qiu Y, Pei L, Jiang R, et al. Nicotinamide riboside attenuates alcohol induced liver injuries via activation of SirT1/PGC-1α/mitochondrial biosynthesis pathway. Redox Biol. 2018;17:89–98.
31. Bota AB, Simmons JG, Dibattista A, Wilson K. Critical review carnitine in alcohol use disorders: a scoping review, vol. 45; 2021. p. 666.

32. Marí M, de Gregorio E, de Dios C, Roca-Agujetas V, Cucarull B, Tutusaus A. et al. Mitochondrial Glutathione: Recent Insights and Role in Disease. Available from: www.mdpi.com/journal/antioxidants
33. Remigante A, Yang YM, Cho YE, Hwang S. Crosstalk between oxidative stress and inflammatory liver injury in the pathogenesis of alcoholic liver disease; 2022. https://doi.org/10.3390/ijms23020774.
34. Wunder C, Weber C, Paulke A, Koelzer SC, Holz F, Toennes SW. Assay of ethanol and congener alcohols in serum and beverages by headspace gas chromatography/mass spectrometry. MethodsX [Internet]. 2021. Aug 1 [cited 2022 Sep 9]; Available from: https://www.ncbi.nlm.nih.gov/pmc/articles/PMC8563810/pdf/main.pdf;8:101563.
35. Fernando H, Victoria R, Ayda E. Determinación de congéneres en alcohol extra neutro rectificado empleado en la elaboración de bebidas alchohólicas. 2015;13:28–37.
36. Rohsenow DJ, Howland J, Arnedt JT, Almeida AB, Greece J, Minsky S, et al. Intoxication with bourbon versus vodka: effects on hangover, sleep, and next-day neurocognitive performance in young adults. Alcohol Clin Exp Res. 2010;34(3):509–18.
37. Wigand P, Blettner M, Saloga J, Decker H. Prävalenz der Weinunverträglichkeit. Dtsch Arztebl Int. 2012;109(25):437–44.
38. Guo R, Jun R. Alcohol and acetaldehyde in public health: from marvel to menace. Int J Environ Res Public Health. MDPI. 2010;7:1285–301.
39. Mizumoto A, Ohashi S, Hirohashi K, Amanuma Y, Matsuda T, Muto M. Molecular sciences molecular mechanisms of acetaldehyde-mediated carcinogenesis in squamous epithelium. 2017;. Available from: www.mdpi.com/journal/ijms
40. Ghosh A, Mahintamani T, Balhara YPS, Roub FE, Basu D, Subodh BN, et al. Disulfiram ethanol reaction with alcohol-based hand sanitizer: an exploratory study. Alcohol Alcohol. 2021;56(1):42–6.
41. Álvarez FJ. Alcohol y alergia, vol. 10. Trastornos Adictivos. Ediciones Doyma, S.L; 2008. p. 75–6.
42. Adams KE, Rans TS. Adverse reactions to alcohol and alcoholic beverages. Ann Allergy Asthma Immunol. 2013;111:439–45.
43. Vasconcelos MJ, Badas J, Bartolomé B, Coimbra A, Silva D. Beer allergy: when malt is the culprit. Ann Allergy Asthma Immunol. 2019;123(2):211–213.e1.
44. Pita JS, Sousa N, Bartolome B, Loureiro C, Bom AT. Beer: an uncommon cause of anaphylaxis. BMJ Case Rep. 2019;12(1)
45. Brussino L, Nicola S, Giorgis V, Rolla G. Beer anaphylaxis due to coriander as hidden allergen. BMJ Case Rep. 2018;2018
46. German-Sanchez A, Alonso-Llamazares A, Garcia-Gonzalez F, Matala-Ahmed B, Bartolome-Zavala B, Antepara-Ercoreca I. Allergy to beer and wine caused by Saccharomyces cerevisiae in a patient sensitized to fungi. J Investigat Allergol Clin Immunol ESMON Publicidad SA. 2022;32:311–3.
47. Gonzalez-Quintela A, Gomez-Rial J, Valcarcel C, Campos J, Sanz ML, Linneberg A, et al. Immunoglobulin-E reactivity to wine glycoproteins in heavy drinkers. Alcohol. 2011;45(2):113–22.
48. Navarro LA, Peláez A, de La Torre F, Burillo T, Megías JM, Martínez J. Epidemiological factors on hymenoptera venom allergy in a Spanish adult population [Internet]. J Investig Allergol Clin Immunol. 2007;77. Available from: www.nejm.org
49. Mirijello A, Sestito L, Antonelli M, Gasbarrini A, Addolorato G. Identification and management of acute alcohol intoxication. Eur J Intern Med. 2022;108:1.
50. Mora TM. Revisión bibliográfica intoxicación alcohólica resumen. 2016;33:2.
51. D'Angelo A, Petrella C, Greco A, Ralli M, Vitali M, Giovagnoli R, et al. Acute alcohol intoxication: a clinical overview, vol. 173. Clinica Terapeutica. Societa Editrice Universo; 2022. p. 280–91.
52. Elsevier. Acute ethanol toxicity terminology clinical clarification [Internet]. 2019. Available from: https://health.gov/dietaryguidelines/2015/guidelines/appendix-9/

53. Burgess HJ, Rizvydeen M, Kikyo F, Kebbeh N, Tan M, Roecklein KA, et al. Sleep and circadian differences between light and heavy adult alcohol drinkers. Alcohol Clin Exp Res. 2022;46:1181–91.
54. de Sousa A. Disulfiram its use in alcohol dependence and other disorders.
55. LoVerde D, Iweala OI, Eginli A, Krishnaswamy G. Anaphylaxis, vol. 153. Chest. Elsevier Inc; 2018. p. 528–43.
56. Schroder JN, Branch MS. Mallory Weiss syndrome. Gastrointestinal bleeding: a practical approach to diagnosis and management [Internet]. 2021 Dec 12 [cited 2022 Sep 16];79–84. Available from: https://www.ncbi.nlm.nih.gov/books/NBK538190/
57. Rumgay H, Murphy N, Ferrari P, Soerjomataram I. Alcohol and cancer: epidemiology and biological mechanisms. 2021 https://doi.org/10.3390/nu13093173.
58. Palmer BF, Clegg DJ. Electrolyte disturbances in patients with chronic alcohol-use disorder. N Engl J Med. 2017;377(14):1368–77.
59. Kandi S, Deshpande N, Rao P, Ramana K, v. Article alcoholism and its relation to hypoglycemia-an overview alcoholism and its relation to hypoglycemia—an overview. Am J Med Stud [Internet]. 2014;2(3):46–9. Available from: http://pubs.sciepub.com/ajms/2/3/2
60. Chatterjee K, Fernandes AB, Goyal S, Shanker S. Central pontine myelinolysis in a case of alcohol dependence syndrome. Ind Psychiatry J [Internet]. 2015;24:198. [cited 2022 Sep 17]. PMCID: PMC4866352

Chapter 5
Acute Interstitial Nephritis

María Mercedes Capotondo, Gustavo Aroca-Martínez, and Carlos Guido Musso

Introduction

Acute Interstitial nephritis (AIN) is a frequent cause of acute kidney injury (AKI) diagnosed in 13–20% of biopsies performed in patients with AKI, so it should be suspected mainly in patients affected by polypharmacy [1, 2]. Globally it is estimated that AIN accounts for 15–20% of AKI cases [3]. The true incidence of this condition is in fact unknown because published studies on AIN retrospectively analyze the data from kidney biopsy (gold standard) records in patients suffering from AKI, not taking into account those patients in whom AIN diagnosis was clinically performed. Thus, it seems that AIN incidence is underestimated since this disease occurs very frequently in frail older patients in whom renal biopsy is usually not performed. The prevalence of biopsy-documented AIN ranges from 0.5 to 2.6% of all renal biopsies, but in an AKI setting, some retrospectively analyzed registries have documented AIN in 5–18% of all kidney biopsies, and drug-induced AIN (DI-AIN) as the third cause of AKI in hospitalized patients [4, 5]. DI-AIN prevalence is high in older individuals mainly due to their high risk of presenting polypharmacy [6].

M. M. Capotondo
Department of Internal Medicine, Hospital Italiano de Buenos Aires, Buenos Aires, Argentina
e-mail: maria.capotondo@hospitalitaliano.org.ar

G. Aroca-Martínez
Faculty of Health Sciences, Universidad Simón Bolívar, Barranquilla, Atlántico, Colombia

C. G. Musso (✉)
Department of Internal Medicine, Hospital Italiano de Buenos Aires, Buenos Aires, Argentina

Faculty of Health Sciences, Universidad Simón Bolívar, Barranquilla, Atlántico, Colombia
e-mail: carlos.musso@hospitalitaliano.org.ar

M. G. Múnera Gómez et al. (eds.), *Allergies, Poisoning and Intolerance to Common Substances*, https://doi.org/10.1007/978-3-031-93658-6_5

AIN Pathophysiology and Etiology

DI-AIN is a dose-independent type IV hypersensitivity immune-allergic reaction that occurs in the renal parenchyma after exposure to different drugs and is characterized by an interstitial infiltrate composed predominantly of T lymphocytes, without significant deposition of immunoglobulins or complement [7]. The drug possibly acts as an allergen or lowers immunological tolerance [1]. In a recent analysis, two possible genomic regions associated with AIN susceptibility were identified, so there could be a genetic basis that predisposes to suffering from this condition [8]. AIN inducing mechanism can be unknown (idiopathic AIN) or it can be caused by drugs, autoimmune diseases, or infections, although DI-AIN is its predominant etiology. Even though practically almost all drugs can cause AIN, antibiotics, non-steroidal anti-inflammatory agents, and proton pump inhibitors represent the majority of them [6].

DI-AIN represents almost two thirds of all AIN cases, although other underlying systemic diseases may also be involved [2, 7]. In turn, 80–90% of DI-AINs have antibiotics, non-steroidal anti-inflammatory agents (NSAIDs), and proton pump inhibitors (PPIs) as their etiology, although immune checkpoint inhibitors (ICIs) have gained increasing attention as a cause of AIN [6].

Allopurinol, diuretics, phenytoin, and H2-receptor antagonists are other known AIN causes [9]. ICIs have recently emerged as an important cause of AIN, which frequently presents as AKI insidiously with a subacute increase in serum creatinine levels and minimal symptoms or urinary abnormalities. Histopathological confirmation of AIN by ICI is usually necessary, delays diagnosis, and has a variable prognosis with 30% of patients requiring dialysis and 40–60% progressing to CKD [2].

A particular case occurs when the patient presents recurrent episodes of AIN (R-AIN). In these patients, it is necessary to look for an underlying etiology different from DI-AIN, such as systemic disease: Sjogren's syndrome, sarcoidosis, light chain gammopathy, or tubulo-interstitial nephritis and uveitis (TINU) syndrome. Therefore, the diagnosis of R-AIN should prompt physicians to look for systemic causes of AIN [7].

The long-term use of PPIs is associated with some renal adverse effects, such as AKI, AIN, chronic kidney disease (CKD), end-stage renal disease (ESRD), and hypomagnesemia secondary to tubular loss. It is believed that the accumulation of PPIs or their metabolites in the tubulo-interstitium could trigger a cell-mediated immune response that could cause AKI, interstitial fibrosis, and/or tubular atrophy. In addition, prolonged use of PPIs generates hypomagnesemia that could result in endothelial cell dysfunction, and consequently in kidney disease progression [10].

The PubMed data on the safety of amoxicillin (AMX) use have recently been reviewed, as although its use for infection prophylaxis and treatment is widely spread, and it is considered to be a relatively safe antibiotic, several reports suggest a risk of nephrotoxicity. AMX nephrotoxicity may be due to different pathophysiological mechanisms, such as type IV hypersensitivity reaction (AIN) or intratubular and/or urinary tract precipitation (AMX crystal nephropathy) [11].

Regarding ICIs, they are widely used in the treatment of many cancers and currently represent the standard of care for multiple malignancies. They work by enhancing the immune response of T cells to attack cancer cells. However, there are important renal immunity-related adverse events (IRAEs) associated with ICI. AIN is the most frequent renal IRAE, although it can also frequently cause glomerular damage and electrolyte disturbances. It is hypothesized that T cells could potentially lose their tolerance to native kidney cells, causing AIN or glomerulonephritis (GN). It has been reported that an adverse drug interaction (second hit) represented by the appearance of drug-induced hypersensitivity to ICI in the presence of PPI, NSAIDs, or vitamin K antagonists, which can potentiate ICI-related immune adverse events. These drugs are thought to act as foreign antigens or haptens, triggering an immune response. In this sense, it has been reported that 70% of patients suffering from ICI-induced AKI had been exposed to other AIN-inducing drugs, mostly PPIs [12]. Moreover, being under treatment with PPIs is a risk factor for AIN due to ICI therapy. The positive staining for PD1 and PD-L1 correlates with cases of AIN caused by ICIs [3]. AIN is a late adverse effect of ICIs, with a median time to AKI onset after ICI onset of 16 weeks. There are different classes of ICIs, the main ones being anti-CTLA4 and anti-PD-1. Renal damage by CTLA4 antagonists occurs 6–12 weeks after cancer treatment, while PD-1 antagonists can damage the kidney only after 6–8 months.

Furthermore, renal damage mediated by anti-CTLA4 is more severe compared to anti-PD-1, which is probably due to a more precise spectrum of T-cell activation mediated by PD-1 blockade compared to CTLA4 [12].

Finally, the AIN cause seems to be changing, and PPIs are beginning to play an important role in causing this renal condition, so there must be a high index of suspicion since delaying the suspension of the offending drug and the start of steroid treatment negatively affects the recovery of kidney function. 70% of AIN cases are associated with drugs, 20% with autoimmune diseases, and 4% with infections. DI-AIN is usually caused by antibiotics in 49%, PPIs in 14%, and NSAIDs in 11%, being the top 3 AIN-inducing drugs: omeprazole (12%), amoxicillin (8%), and ciprofloxacin (8%). Patients with PPI-induced AIN were older, less symptomatic, with a longer duration of drug exposure, and longer delays in obtaining a renal biopsy and starting steroid treatment than patients with antibiotic or NSAID-induced AIN [13].

Clinical Presentation

In most cases, AIN-related symptoms are nonspecific and include nausea, vomiting, and general malaise, although many patients are asymptomatic. The classic triad is characterized by fever, maculopapular rash, and eosinophilia and is associated with exposure to antibiotics not currently used such as methicillin, but less symptomatic forms characterized by longer intervals between drug exposure and symptom onset are becoming more frequent, making it difficult to identify the causative agent [6, 7].

The most common presentation is asymptomatic elevation of serum creatinine and urea levels. In DI-AIN, non-oliguric AKI is the main renal manifestation, and non-nephrotic tubular proteinuria is usually present (range: 0.7 to 1.5 g/24 h). Additionally, the incidence of nephrotic syndrome seems to be low and represents around 2.53% of patients. Patients with NSAID-induced AIN present higher levels of proteinuria than other types of DI-AIN, and even nephrotic proteinuria can be documented. The AIN extrarenal manifestations (rash, fever, and eosinophilia), commonly observed in antibiotic-associated AIN, are characteristically absent in NSAID-induced AIN. As renal damage progresses, nonspecific AKI symptoms of any cause appear, such as malaise, anorexia, nausea and vomiting, and flank pain, as well as hematuria with or without oliguria (pseudo-nephritic syndrome). The classic triad (rash, fever, and eosinophilia) is present in only 5–10% of cases, and when present, the rash is usually a truncal maculopapular morbilliform rash. The triad is characteristic of methicillin-related AIN, and this antibiotic is not currently used. Another form of presentation is the presence of AIN associated with bilateral uveitis (TINU), but this is a rare presentation, more frequent in adolescent females; the median age is 19 years, and females are more commonly affected than males (2:1). Both renal and ocular disease can be asymptomatic, may not manifest simultaneously, and have independent progressions. Kidney disease manifests as AKI and can cause permanent kidney failure. Uveitis can also progress and become chronic. The classic presentation triad induced by antibiotics and accompanied by obvious manifestations of hypersensitivity such as rash, eosinophilia, and fever, has been largely replaced by frequent oligosymptomatic presentations in older patients, often associated with the use of NSAIDs and PPIs, requiring a high index of suspicion [6, 14–16]. It is worth mentioning that, as it happens with other conditions in older individuals, AIN can usually present with the appearance of geriatric syndromes (geriatric giants), such as confusional syndrome, gait disorders, falls, immobility syndrome, as well as urinary and/or fecal incontinence [17].

The presentation form of ICI-induced AIN also differs from the presentation form of classical AIN. Patients diagnosed with ICI-induced AIN have lower serum creatinine levels at diagnosis, milder AKI but slower creatinine improvement, higher urine and white blood cell counts, and a longer latency period after initiation of the offending drug compared with patients with AIN secondary to other etiologies. This differential evolution may be due to differences in their pathophysiological mechanisms [18].

In a study where AIN was evaluated in the pediatric population, it was observed that it is an infrequent cause of AKI in children, and of the 24 patients evaluated, 37.5% were associated with TINU syndrome, 16.7% were associated with an autoimmune disease, 16.7% were probably drug-induced and 37.5% had an unclear etiology [19].

The time interval between the start of the offending drug and the AIN episode can vary, being short in the case of beta-lactams and cephalosporins, occurring after prolonged exposure as in the case of AIN induced by PPIs or NSAIDs, or presenting after even longer latency period as in the case of ICI-AIN, as well as a slower decrease in serum creatinine levels after treatment. Rifampicin-induced AIN usually occurs when the antibiotic is reintroduced after a time interval, and the latency period may be as short as 1 day. Methicillin-associated AKI is early onset (after a few days to weeks) and is associated with rash, fever, and eosinophilia, with fever being the most common feature and arthralgias the least common. Rifampicin-induced AIN manifests as headache, chills, dark-colored urine without hematuria, and oliguric AKI [6].

AIN Diagnosis

The definitive AIN diagnosis is given by a renal biopsy. However, renal biopsy is not always performed since, on one hand, the affected patients are frequently fragile with a high risk of complications, and on the other hand, AIN manifests with slight serum creatinine elevation, and its diagnosis is assumed without a renal biopsy. AIN is histologically characterized by an extensive interstitial infiltrate mainly composed of lymphocytes and monocytes. There may be tubulitis and tubular degeneration signs, such as loss of the brush border, epithelium flattening, and shedding of cells toward the tubular lumen. Urinalysis shows sterile pyuria in up to two-thirds of cases, leukocyte casts (3–14%), and hematuria. The presence of microscopic hematuria is associated with a more severe disease and worse renal outcomes. One-third of patients with AIN present red blood cell casts, probably related to disruption of interstitial blood vessels and consequent leakage of erythrocytes into the tubular lumen. The diagnosis of DI-AIN requires a high index of suspicion, but a renal biopsy is required to confirm the diagnosis. Although eosinophiluria has been considered a specific characteristic of AIN, the presence of eosinophiluria in the urinary sediment is a nonspecific and unreliable finding since it can be seen in many other renal diseases such as urinary tract infections, acute tubular necrosis, and glomerulonephritis [6].

AIN Treatment

In DI-AIN, treatment consists of discontinuing the inducing drug as soon as possible, and unless a rapid recovery of renal function is observed (after 5–7 days since interruption), several studies support that a course of glucocorticoids should be started. Corticosteroids used early would reduce the inflammatory infiltrate of the renal interstitium, thus preventing the risk of later fibrosis [2, 6].

Although glucocorticoid therapy is known to be used frequently if there is no renal improvement despite drug discontinuation, its use is controversial as data from randomized controlled trials is not available, and regimens with steroid treatment are not standardized. Some case series and small retrospective studies have shown the benefit of using corticosteroids in DI-AIN, but others have not. However, there is a rationale for glucocorticoid therapy in DI-AIN based on the fact that glucocorticoids block cytokine production and inhibit a key proinflammatory transcription factor, NF-kB, which has an essential role in promoting renal inflammation. A few days after the initial tubulointerstitial inflammation, fibroblast-mediated profibrotic processes and epithelial-mesenchymal transformation are activated, resulting in interstitial collagen deposition, irreversible tubular atrophy, and tubulo-interstitial fibrosis (TIF). The use of corticosteroids early in the course of the disease can prevent TIF by attenuating the initial pro-inflammatory pathways. However there are retrospective studies that found no benefit from the use of glucocorticoids in DI-AIN, and these results could have several possible explanations, such as the selection bias in these retrospective studies that would favor the results in those who do not receive treatment with steroids, since the steroids would be tested in patients who do not improve with discontinuation of the drug, and furthermore, the delay in the initiation of steroid treatment and the presence of a higher grade of TIF in the renal biopsy would predict a lower response to steroids. Timely therapy with corticosteroids could allow rapid and complete recovery of renal function and reduce the risk of residual CKD. A reasonable short course of high-dose steroid treatment (2–3 weeks) followed by a taper over the next 6–8 weeks is a reasonable approach although when the offending drug is an ICI, a longer treatment (3–6 months) and a slower decrease in corticosteroids may be required. There are no advantages of intravenous protocols over high-dose oral steroids [1].

González et al., in a multicenter retrospective study of 61 cases of biopsy-proven DI-AIN, demonstrated that at 18 months, the glucocorticoid group had lower serum creatinine, more complete renal recovery, and less dialysis dependency compared with controls without glucocorticoids, although observing significant adverse effects of steroids. A delay in starting treatment was associated with poor renal recovery. This study suggested that rapid initiation of glucocorticoids within the first 7 days in patients with DI-AIN may improve renal recovery and reduce TIF and the risk of future CKD [20].

Raza et al. demonstrated that the use of corticosteroids was associated with lower creatinine values and a lower risk of requiring dialysis, although the latter was not statistically significant [21].

Muriithi et al. who evaluated renal outcomes 6 months after biopsy in 83 patients with DI-AIN treated with steroids (versus 12 controls) and demonstrated that prolonged drug exposure and delayed initiation of glucocorticoid therapy were correlated with suboptimal renal recovery [13].

There are no studies in the literature on the prospective recruitment of patients with DI-AIN that allow guiding the treatment of this condition, and the existing studies are heterogeneous and of low quality of evidence and cannot be meta-analyzed [22].

Regarding ICI-AIN treatment, it consists of temporary cessation of immunotherapy, corticosteroid treatment, and discontinuation of AIN-associated medications, such as PPIs and NSAIDs. Treatment should be started as soon as the diagnosis of AIN is strongly suspected, and early initiation of corticosteroids within 3 days of

ICI-AIN diagnosis was associated with greater odds of renal recovery compared with late initiation. The usual recommended corticosteroid regimen is to initially treat stage 1 or 2 AKIN with 0.8 to 1.0 mg/kg of prednisone up to 60 mg daily for 1–2 weeks, followed by a gradual taper over 4–6 weeks. For stage 3 AKIN, a pulsed-dose intravenous corticosteroid followed by treatment with oral prednisone is preferred. The duration of treatment with corticosteroids and the speed of their reduction are not defined [12, 23].

A group at the Massachusetts General Hospital Cancer Center developed a clinical protocol for rapid tapering of corticosteroids. They compared patients treated with a protocol of rapid reduction in 3 weeks with a standard protocol of reduction in corticosteroid doses in 6 weeks, showing equivalent renal recovery between the two groups. However, Manohar et al. found that patients treated with a rapid taper over 4 weeks had a higher risk of AKI recurrence [24, 25].

Even when AIN is suspected to be secondary to drugs, it is often difficult to identify the putative drug due to the large list of possible drugs suspected to be involved in DI-AIN, due to polypharmacy especially those with chronic diseases and advanced age, who are at particularly high risk for DI-AIN due to their frailty, the variable time from drug exposure to AKI, the lack of accurate screening methods to discriminate the offending drug, and the increasingly widespread use of over-the-counter medications such as NSAIDs or PPIs [6].

In a biopsy-proven multicenter study of DI-AIN, González et al. demonstrated a significant correlation between delayed initiation of corticosteroid treatment and incomplete recovery of renal function [20].

In another retrospective study reviewing the results of renal biopsies from a period of 12 years, Clarkson et al. did not detect a statistically significant difference in the result, as determined by serum creatinine, among those patients who did or did not receive corticosteroids, one month, 6, or 12 months after presentation [26].

In a systematic review of the literature that included studies comparing the effects of corticosteroid treatment versus non-corticosteroid treatment, considerable heterogeneity was observed, corticosteroid treatment was poorly defined, the risk of bias was high in all domains, and it was concluded that the limited evidence does not support the use of corticosteroids in the treatment of DI-AIN and that larger, well-designed trials are needed to help to guide the clinical management of this condition [27].

Fernández-Juárez et al. carried out a retrospective study of 182 patients with biopsy-proven DI-AIN from 13 Spanish centers. The duration of treatment with corticosteroids was evaluated, and the recovery of renal function was measured with serum creatinine at 6 months. The longer treatment time (>8 weeks) did not show benefits compared to a 3-week steroid treatment in terms of recovery of renal function. Late initiation of steroid treatment and the presence of >50% interstitial fibrosis in the renal biopsy sample were associated with a 6-month serum creatinine level greater than 75% compared to baseline values. Forty-eight percent of patients were treated with intravenous pulsed corticosteroids prior to oral administration. Neither the initial dose of corticosteroids nor the duration of treatment (3 or more than 8 weeks) seems to influence the recovery of renal function [28].

In a comparative study evaluating oral corticosteroid therapy with pulsed intravenous corticosteroid therapy followed by oral corticosteroids, early steroid therapy, both oral and pulsed, was shown to be equally effective in drug-induced AIN [29].

In conclusion, since the evidence in the literature comes from retrospective studies, the treatment of AIN continues to be a challenge. However, there is evidence on the use of corticosteroids for the treatment of this entity when it is started quickly [6].

The quality of the evidence of the studies that evaluate the use or non-use of corticosteroids is low, and it is important to carry out well-designed randomized control trials or large observational studies that provide high-quality evidence, the definition of the most appropriate corticosteroid regimen, and the search for non-invasive biomarkers to replace or complement renal biopsy [30].

There is an ongoing multicenter, prospective, randomized, controlled, open-label study that includes incident adult patients with biopsy-proven AIN, in which patients will be randomized 1:1 to one of 2 treatment regimens: treatment with prednisolone (60 mg daily and reduced for 8 weeks) and a control group. It is planned to include and follow up with 110 patients for 1 year. The researchers will assess renal function at 3 and 6 months and the need for renal replacement therapy. Trial registration: ClinicalTrials.gov identifier NCT04376216 [31].

Conclusion

Acute interstitial nephritis is a frequent cause of acute kidney injury, so it should always be suspected, especially in patients with polypharmacy, since its main variant is drug-induced. Its certain diagnosis is through renal biopsy, although it is frequently not performed because this condition usually affects frail older individuals. To date, there are no quality prospective studies to define the best therapeutic regimen, although early treatment with corticosteroids seems to be beneficial.

Glossary

Glossary of Acronyms

AAAAI American Academy of Allergy, Asthma, and Immunology
ADH Alcohol Dehydrogenase
AIN Acute Interstitial Nephritis
ALDH Aldehyde Dehydrogenase
Cd Cadmium
CYP450 Cytochrome P450
EtOH Ethanol
GABA Gamma-Aminobutyric Acid

Hg Mercury
IgE Immunoglobulin E
LI Lactose Intolerance
NAD Nicotinamide Adenine Dinucleotide
NAD+ Nicotinamide Adenine Dinucleotide (Oxidized Form)
NADH Nicotinamide Adenine Dinucleotide (Reduced Form)
NSAIDs Non-Steroidal Anti-Inflammatory Drugs
PPIs Proton Pump Inhibitors
REM Rapid Eye Movement
SPT Skin Prick Test
Th2 Type 2 Helper T cells
Vd Volume of Distribution

Glossary of Terms

Acute Intoxication Rapid onset of symptoms following exposure to a toxic substance.

Atopic Dermatitis A type of inflammation of the skin (eczema), often associated with allergies.

BAL (British Anti-Lewisite) A chelating agent used in the treatment of heavy metal poisoning.

Cadmium (Cd) A heavy metal with no biological function in humans, often associated with industrial pollution.

Chelation Therapy Treatment that involves the administration of chelating agents to remove heavy metals from the body.

Chronic Exposure Prolonged exposure to a toxic substance, often leading to long-term health effects.

Contact Dermatitis Inflammation of the skin caused by contact with certain substances.

Dermal Absorption The process by which a substance passes through the skin and into the body.

DMPS (2,3-Dimercapto-1-propanesulfonic acid) A chelating agent used to treat heavy metal poisoning.

DMSA (2,3-Dimercaptosuccinic acid) A chelating agent used to treat heavy metal poisoning.

Elemental Mercury (Hg0) The pure form of mercury, which is liquid at room temperature and highly toxic.

IgE (Immunoglobulin E) An antibody associated with allergic reactions.

Inhalation Exposure The intake of substances through breathing.

Mercury (Hg) A highly toxic heavy metal that exists in elemental, inorganic, and organic forms.

Metallothioneins Proteins that bind heavy metals and aid in their detoxification.

Methylmercury (Me-Hg) A highly toxic form of mercury found in certain fish and seafood.

Nickel (Ni) A heavy metal commonly associated with allergic reactions and contact dermatitis.

Non-Essential Heavy Metals Metals that have no beneficial role in biological systems and are toxic even at low concentrations.

Patch Test A diagnostic tool used to identify allergic reactions to various substances.

Thimerosal An organic mercury compound used as a preservative in vaccines and other products.

References

1. Donati A, Krishnan N. Should corticosteroids be used to treat biopsy-proven drug-induced acute interstitial nephritis?: PRO. Kidney360. 2022;3(8):1306–9.
2. Caravaca-Fontán F, Fernández-Juárez G, Praga M. Acute kidney injury in interstitial nephritis. Curr Opin Crit Care. 2019;25(6):558–64.
3. Casals J, Acosta Y, Caballero G, Morantes L, Zamora C, Xipell M, et al. Differentiating acute interstitial nephritis from immune checkpoint inhibitors from other causes. Kidney Int Rep. 2022;8(3):672–5.
4. Praga M, Sevillano A, Auñón P, González E. Changes in the aetiology, clinical presentation and management of acute interstitial nephritis, an increasingly common cause of acute kidney injury. Nephrol Dial Transplant Off Publ Eur Dial Transpl Assoc—Eur Ren Assoc. 2015;30(9):1472–9.
5. Raghavan R, Eknoyan G. Acute interstitial nephritis—a reappraisal and update. Clin Nephrol. 2014;82(3):149–62.
6. Sanchez-Alamo B, Cases-Corona C, Fernandez-Juarez G. Facing the challenge of drug-induced acute interstitial nephritis. Nephron. 2023;147(2):78–90.
7. Caravaca-Fontán F, Shabaka A, Sánchez-Álamo B, de Lorenzo A, Díaz M, Blasco M, et al. Recurrent acute interstitial nephritis: what lies beneath. Clin Kidney J. 2021;14(1):197–204.
8. Zhou XJ, Su T, Xie J, Xie QH, Wang LZ, Hu Y, et al. Genome-wide association study in acute Tubulointerstitial nephritis. J Am Soc Nephrol JASN. 2023;34(5):895–908.
9. Medication-Induced Interstitial Nephritis in the 21st Century—ClinicalKey [Internet]. [cited 2023 May 29]. Available from: https://www-clinicalkey-es.hospitalitaliano.idm.oclc.org/#!/content/journal/1-s2.0-S1548559516301446
10. Maideen NMP. Adverse effects associated with long-term use of proton pump inhibitors. Chonnam Med J. 2023;59(2):115–27.
11. Garnier AS, Drablier G, Briet M, Augusto JF. Nephrotoxicity of amoxicillin and third-generation Cephalosporins: an updated review. Drug Saf. 2023;46:715.
12. Rao Ullur A, Côté G, Pelletier K, Kitchlu A. Immunotherapy in oncology and the kidneys: a clinical review of the evaluation and management of kidney immune-related adverse events. Clin Kidney J. 2023;16(6):939–51.
13. Muriithi AK, Leung N, Valeri AM, Cornell LD, Sethi S, Fidler ME, et al. Biopsy-proven acute interstitial nephritis, 1993–2011: a case series. Am J Kidney Dis Off J Natl Kidney Found. 2014;64(4):558–66.
14. Interstitial Nephritis—ClinicalKey [Internet]. [cited 2023 Mar 17]. Available from: https://www-clinicalkey-es.hospitalitaliano.idm.oclc.org/#!/content/derived_clinical_overview/76-s2.0-B9780323755733005072
15. Southgate G, Clarke P, Harmer MJ. Renal outcomes in tubulointerstitial nephritis and uveitis (TINU) syndrome: a systematic review and meta-analysis. J Nephrol. 2023;36(2):507–19.

16. Amaro D, Carreño E, Steeples LR, Oliveira-Ramos F, Marques-Neves C, Leal I. Tubulointerstitial nephritis and uveitis (TINU) syndrome: a review. Br J Ophthalmol. 2020;104(6):742–7.
17. Musso CG, Jauregui JR, Macias-Nuñez JF, Covic A. Frailty in kidney disease. Cham: Springer; 2019.
18. Draibe JB, García-Carro C, Martinez-Valenzuela L, Agraz I, Fulladosa X, Bolufer M, et al. Acute tubulointerstitial nephritis induced by checkpoint inhibitors versus classical acute tubulointerstitial nephritis: are they the same disease? Clin Kidney J. 2021;14(3):884–90.
19. Biederman LE, Conces M, Shenoy A. Acute interstitial nephritis in the pediatric population: a review of etiologic associations, histologic findings, and clinical outcome. Pediatr Dev Pathol Off J Soc Pediatr Pathol Paediatr Pathol Soc. 2023;26(1):13–7.
20. González E, Gutiérrez E, Galeano C, Chevia C, de Sequera P, Bernis C, et al. Early steroid treatment improves the recovery of renal function in patients with drug-induced acute interstitial nephritis. Kidney Int. 2008;73(8):940–6.
21. Raza MN, Hadid M, Keen CE, Bingham C, Salmon AHJ. Acute tubulointerstitial nephritis, treatment with steroid and impact on renal outcomes. Nephrol Carlton Vic. 2012;17(8):748–53.
22. Gallagher MP, Kotwal S. Should corticosteroids be used to treat biopsy-proven drug-induced acute interstitial nephritis?: CON. Kidney360. 2022;3(8):1310–3.
23. Capotondo M, Aroca Martínez G, Specterman S, Musso CG. Acute kidney injury in oncology. In: Rezaei N, editor. Interdisciplinary cancer research. Springer; 2023. https://doi.org/10.1007/16833_2023_162.
24. Lee MD, Seethapathy H, Strohbehn IA, Zhao SH, Boland GM, Fadden R, et al. Rapid corticosteroid taper versus standard of care for immune checkpoint inhibitor induced nephritis: a single-center retrospective cohort study. J Immunother Cancer. 2021;9(4):e002292.
25. Manohar S, Ghamrawi R, Chengappa M, Goksu BNB, Kottschade L, Finnes H, et al. Acute interstitial nephritis and checkpoint inhibitor therapy. Kidney360. 2020;1(1):16–24.
26. Clarkson MR, Giblin L, O'Connell FP, O'Kelly P, Walshe JJ, Conlon P, et al. Acute interstitial nephritis: clinical features and response to corticosteroid therapy. Nephrol Dial Transplant Off Publ Eur Dial Transpl Assoc—Eur Ren Assoc. 2004;19(11):2778–83.
27. Quinto LR, Sukkar L, Gallagher M. Effectiveness of corticosteroid compared with non-corticosteroid therapy for the treatment of drug-induced acute interstitial nephritis: a systematic review. Intern Med J. 2019;49(5):562–9.
28. Fernandez-Juarez G, Perez JV, Caravaca-Fontán F, Quintana L, Shabaka A, Rodríguez E, et al. Duration of treatment with corticosteroids and recovery of kidney function in acute interstitial nephritis. Clin J Am Soc Nephrol CJASN. 2018;13(12):1851–8.
29. Ramachandran R, Kumar K, Nada R, Jha V, Gupta KL, Kohli HS. Drug-induced acute interstitial nephritis: a clinicopathological study and comparative trial of steroid regimens. Indian J Nephrol. 2015;25(5):281–6.
30. Praga M, Caravaca-Fontán F. Should corticosteroids be used to treat biopsy-proven drug-induced acute interstitial nephritis? Commentary Kidney360. 2022;3(8):1314–6.
31. Mose FH, Birn H, Hoffmann-Petersen N, Bech JN. Prednisolone treatment in acute interstitial nephritis (PRAISE)—protocol for the randomized controlled trial. BMC Nephrol. 2021;22(1):161.

Chapter 6
Heavy Metal Poisoning and Its Relationship with Allergies

Johana Márquez-Lázaro and Yuliana Emiliani Navarro

Introduction

Heavy metals are elements that naturally occur in the Earth's crust; however, anthropogenic activity has led to drastic changes in their geochemical cycles [1]. These metals are characterized by having a high atomic weight, densities higher than that of water (more than five times), and being difficult to degrade [1, 2]. They are classified into essential and non-essential heavy metals [2]. The former are beneficial for human health and other living beings but can be toxic when concentrations exceed the tolerable limit for organisms [1, 2]; these include zinc, copper, iron, manganese, and cobalt [1, 3].

On the other hand, non-essential heavy metals are toxic to living beings at any concentration, and their presence in the environment derives primarily from mining and industrial activities. This group includes cadmium (Cd), copper (Cu), lead (Pb), mercury (Hg), arsenic (As), and nickel (Ni) [1–3]. It has been demonstrated that the accumulation of these metals can alter the body's metabolic functions in various intricate ways. Additionally, they can accumulate in vital organs such as the liver, heart, kidneys, and brain, disrupting normal biological functioning [1–4].

These metals can enter the body through various routes, including dermal, inhalation, or ingestion. The latter is promoted by increased industrialization processes that have led to their presence in drinking water and victuals such as vegetables, grains, fruits, fish, shellfish, and meat [4]. Furthermore, particulate

J. Márquez-Lázaro (✉)
Research Group TOXSA, Faculty of Health, Corporación Universitaria Rafael Núñez, Cartagena, Colombia
e-mail: johana.marquez@curnvirtual.edu.co

Y. E. Navarro
GINUMED, Faculty of Health, Corporación Universitaria Rafael Núñez, Cartagena, Colombia
e-mail: yemilianin10@curnvirtual.edu.co

M. G. Múnera Gómez et al. (eds.), *Allergies, Poisoning and Intolerance to Common Substances*, https://doi.org/10.1007/978-3-031-93658-6_6

matter present in the environment constitutes an inhalation exposure route for these contaminants, due to its high adsorption capacity that allows it to serve as a transport vehicle from high to low contamination areas [5]. The risk of exposure through these particles lies in their ease of passing through the respiratory system, depositing in the lungs and bronchi, or reaching the bloodstream when they pass through the lung wall [5, 6].

In this kaleidoscopic context, environmental contamination by non-essential heavy metals constitutes a significant health risk factor worldwide [7]. Their presence in the body has been linked to intoxications (acute or chronic) and the development of allergies such as atopic dermatitis, contact allergy, rhinitis, eczema, and food allergy, events that, in most cases, cannot be countered by the body in the short term due to a lack of necessary mechanisms for their biotransformation and subsequent excretion [1, 3, 4]. In this sense, the detoxification carried out by the body occurs progressively, through the binding of metals to accessory proteins such as metallothioneins, calprotectin, and phytochelatins [4].

Therefore, the objective of this chapter is to delve into the deleterious effects of exposure to heavy metals concerning poisoning and allergy promotion. For this, we will focus on nickel, cadmium, and mercury, as their environmental presence has garnered significant public health interest.

Cadmium

Cadmium (Cd) is a heavy metal that has no biological function in the human body. It is found in nature at low concentrations, often combined with minerals such as zinc sulfide, lead, and copper. However, the presence of this metal in the environment is mainly due to anthropogenic activities. The combustion of fossil fuels, leachates generated in landfills, agricultural lands, and mining waste, especially from zinc and lead mines, significantly contribute to cadmium contamination [8, 9].

Additionally, cadmium is widely used as a pigment for borosilicate glass, in the manufacture of Ni-Cd batteries, as a PVC stabilizer, in alloys, and as an anticorrosive for steel in the electroplating industry. Consequently, the presence of this metal in the environment has become ubiquitous, to the extent that it is found in measurable amounts in food, beverages, and air [8–10].

Cadmium is primarily absorbed through the respiratory tract (10–50%) and, to a lesser extent, through the gastrointestinal tract (5–10%). Dermal absorption of this metal is considered relatively rare. Once in the body, Cd is transported to the bloodstream via erythrocytes, albumin, and metallothioneins and then accumulates in the kidneys, liver, and intestines. Excretion occurs slowly through the kidneys, urine, saliva, and breast milk [9, 11, 12]. In this context, the presence of cadmium in the body (intoxication) has been associated with a variety of adverse effects, including renal and hepatic dysfunction, pulmonary edema, testicular damage, osteomalacia, and damage to the adrenal glands and the hematopoietic and immune systems [9]. Moreover, Cd exposure has also been linked to the development of allergies [7, 13].

Cadmium and Poisoning

Cadmium is considered a highly toxic heavy metal, with a half-life in humans ranging from 10 to 33 years. Poisoning from this metal can occur acutely or chronically through inhalation or the consumption of contaminated water and/or food [8, 9].

Inhalatory exposure to Cd generally occurs at the occupational level and in proximity to industrial or mining areas through dust or vapors generated by mining processes. Another significant source associated with this exposure route is tobacco consumption, with cadmium concentrations ranging between 1 and 2 μg [9].

Regarding food, high concentrations of cadmium have been detected in crustaceans, bivalve mollusks, oysters, cephalopods, and crabs, as well as in offal products such as liver and kidney, oilseeds, cocoa beans, and certain wild mushrooms. Plant-derived foods, depending on soil contamination levels, generally contain higher concentrations of Cd than meat, eggs, milk, and dairy products. Among these, rice and wheat, leafy green vegetables, potatoes, carrots, and celery can contain higher concentrations of the metal compared to other plant-based foods. Seafood consumers and vegetarians may be exposed to higher cadmium intake than omnivores, with rice consumption being one of the main routes of cadmium exposure [8, 9, 11, 14].

A historical event related to the consumption of cadmium-contaminated rice occurred in Toyama Prefecture, Japan, where the metal was released from a zinc mine into the Jinzu River, whose waters were used for crop irrigation. Cadmium intoxication resulted in a disease known as Itai-Itai, characterized by severe pain in individuals with spinal and joint lesions [15]. Itai-Itai patients exhibited a wide range of symptoms, such as low bone mineralization, severe skeletal decalcification, a high fracture rate, and distortion of long bones, osteomalacia, intense bone pain, and osteoporosis. Other complications included cough, anemia, and kidney failure [9].

Clinical Manifestations of Cadmium Poisoning

Cadmium toxicity depends on the route, quantity, and rate of exposure. Consequently, poisoning can be acute or chronic, depending on the exposure pathway (Table 6.1). In the case of chronic exposure (low to moderate doses), the following manifestations may occur:

(a) Renal: Characterized by proximal tubulopathy with initially low molecular weight proteinuria, progressing to high molecular weight proteinuria. These events are accompanied by glucosuria, aminoaciduria, phosphaturia, and calciuria. This can affect calcium metabolism, cause calciuria, and inhibit the hydroxylation of vitamin D.
(b) Pulmonary: Obstructive and restrictive syndromes, progressive pulmonary emphysema, and even pulmonary fibrosis.

Table 6.1 Acute and chronic clinical manifestations of cadmium, mercury, and nickel poisoning

Toxic metal	Acute clinical manifestations	Chronic clinical manifestations
Cadmium	Respiratory distress, nausea, vomiting, abdominal pain	Kidney damage, bone fragility, respiratory issues
Mercury	Tremors, insomnia, memory loss, neuromuscular changes	Cognitive impairment, motor dysfunction, kidney damage
Nickel	Dermatitis, nausea, vomiting, abdominal cramps	Respiratory issues, skin allergies, lung fibrosis

(c) Skeletal: Renal damage with hypercalciuria leading to osteomalacia, which presents as symmetrical bone fissures, particularly appearing in the femoral neck. This condition affects postmenopausal women, causing severe pain in the pelvis and lower limbs (Itai-Itai disease).
(d) Cardiovascular: Alterations in the arterial wall and hypertension (occupational exposure).
(e) Hematological: Anemia (iron transport), leukocytosis, and lymphocytosis.
(f) Other: Anosmia, weight loss, fatigue, yellow discoloration of teeth, increased dental caries, and microcytic-hypochromic anemia unresponsive to treatment [9, 11].

Diagnosis of Cadmium Poisoning

The diagnosis is based on the history of exposure and the presence of respiratory complaints (inhalation) or gastroenteritis (acute ingestion) [11]. Cadmium levels in whole blood can confirm recent exposure; normal levels in non-exposed non-smokers are below 1 mcg/L. Very little cadmium is excreted in the urine until it exceeds the binding capacity of the kidneys or causes renal damage. Urinary cadmium values are typically below 1 mcg/g creatinine. Measurements of tubular microproteinuria (beta2-microglobulin, retinol-binding protein, albumin, and metallothionein) are used to monitor the early and toxic effects of cadmium on the kidneys. Other useful laboratory studies include complete blood count, electrolytes, glucose, blood urea nitrogen, creatinine, arterial blood gases or oximetry, and chest X-ray [16].

Treatment of Cadmium Poisoning

Emergency and Support Measures [16]

- Inhalation: Monitor arterial gases and perform a chest X-ray. It is recommended to observe the patient for at least 6–8 h. In case of wheezing and pulmonary edema, treat the patient with conventional procedures. After significant exposure, it is suggested to observe the patient for 1–2 days to rule out late-onset non-cardiogenic pulmonary edema.
- Ingestion: Treat fluid loss caused by gastroenteritis with IV crystalloid fluids.

Specific Drugs and Antidotes [9, 16]

Acute cadmium poisoning from overexposure is generally treated with chelating agents; however, there is insufficient evidence that this therapy is effective. The chelating agents used include EDTA (ethylenediaminetetraacetic acid), BAL (British Anti-Lewisite, dimercaprol), DMSA (2,3-dimercaptosuccinic acid), and DMPS (2,3-dimercapto-1-propanesulfonic acid). Unlike DMSA, DMPS is transported to the intracellular space where it functions as a chelator. DMSA analogs, such as MmDMSA (monomethyl DMSA), MiADMSA (monoisooctyl DMSA), and MchDMSA (monocyclohexyl DMSA), are more effective and safer antidotes for heavy metal poisoning compared to DMSA. BAL, D-penicillamine (DPCN), and EDTA are contraindicated due to the higher risk of renal damage. On the other hand, biologically active natural compounds such as polyphenolic substances, melatonin, carotenoids, quercetin, resveratrol, vitamin E, vitamin C, L-carnitine, and coenzyme Q10 may be useful in preventing adverse health effects resulting from heavy metal exposure, including cadmium.

Decontamination [16]

1. Inhalation: Remove the victim from exposure and administer supplemental oxygen if available.
2. Ingestion: Perform gastric lavage after significant ingestion.
3. Skin and Eyes: Remove contaminated clothing and wash exposed skin with water. Irrigate exposed eyes with plenty of warm water or saline solution.

Cadmium and Allergies

Air pollution plays an important role in the exposure to environmental contaminants from anthropogenic activities, as it contains particulate matter, which serves as a transport vehicle for these contaminants. In this context, cadmium, like other heavy metals, spreads from mining and industrial areas to areas with less influence. Once in contact with people, the particulate matter easily penetrates the respiratory system and deposits in the lungs and bronchi, where the contaminants eventually interact with the immune system, promoting various responses [17]. This effect can also occur through the consumption of contaminated food and water. Under this context, cadmium and the development of allergies have become a topic of interest to the scientific community.

The exact mechanism of cadmium-induced immune response in humans is still in its early stages; however, in vitro and in vivo studies have shown that this metal can directly interact with immune system cells, causing alterations in their state and functionality [18].

Clinical Manifestations of Cadmium-Induced Allergy

Exposure to environments with high levels of cadmium can promote cough, asthma, rhinitis, wheezing, and atopic dermatitis [19, 20]. Prenatal and postnatal exposure to cadmium has become a marker for detecting allergies and associated diseases in children. Thus, environments with high levels of cadmium have been associated with a higher risk of rhinitis in children [7]. During the early and late weeks of gestation, the presence of cadmium has been linked to a higher incidence of pediatric asthma and the presence of atopic dermatitis in six-month-old infants [5, 6, 21, 22].

Additionally, elevated cadmium levels in people living near mining and smelting areas have been negatively associated with low levels of CD14+ monocytes, which can increase the risk of sepsis-related mortality by affecting the function of immune cells [17, 18].

Diagnosis and Treatment of Cadmium-Induced Allergy

Currently, there is no specific diagnosis and treatment for allergic processes mediated by cadmium exposure. However, the available evidence is associated with the metal levels in the blood and the presented allergic symptoms [5–7, 17–22]. To mitigate the effects of cadmium, it is suggested to implement strategies that reduce the environmental levels of this metal.

Mercury

Mercury (Hg) is a highly toxic heavy metal found in nature in elemental (Hg^0), inorganic (Hg^+, Hg^{+2}), and organic (methyl and ethyl mercury) forms. Elemental mercury is liquid at room temperature and can easily evaporate to produce vapor. Mercury vapor is more dangerous than the liquid form. Organic mercury compounds, such as methyl and ethyl mercury (Me-Hg and Et-Hg, respectively), are more toxic than inorganic compounds. Me-Hg is known as a neurotoxin, as it primarily affects the brain [23]. The increasing toxicity order of these forms is defined as Hg0 < Hg2+, Hg + <CH3-Hg [4, 24].

Mercury compounds have many applications in mining, for example, gold extraction, and some industrial processes. In lamp manufacturing plants, Hg is used in the production of fluorescent bulbs, and in dentistry, it has been used for the preparation of dental amalgams. Me-Hg and Et-Hg have been used as fungicides, and currently, thimerosal, another organic compound, is used as a preservative in multi-dose vaccine vials [25, 26].

Due to its biogeochemical cycle, mercury can interconvert into its three forms. Hg^0 present in the atmosphere settles in water, where microorganisms transform it into Me-Hg, which is ingested by smaller creatures and eventually consumed by larger fish. Fish at the top of the food chain, such as tuna, swordfish, or shark, tend to concentrate a considerable amount of this compound in their tissues [23, 27].

Under this context, people can be exposed to mercury through the inhalation of Hg^0 vapors from dental amalgams, mining, and accidental spills (thermometers, barometers, thermostats) and by ingesting seafood and fish (freshwater and saltwater) that bioaccumulate Me-Hg [25].

Toxicokinetics of Mercury

Hg^0 vapor is easily absorbed from the lungs (80%) and distributed throughout the body. Hg^0 can cross the blood-brain barrier and the placenta, making its neurotoxicity higher than that of inorganic Hg, which crosses membranes at a slower rate. Hg^0 is oxidized in the body to produce Hg^{2+}. Liquid Hg^0 is slightly absorbed in the gastrointestinal tract and does not appear to be toxic. Inorganic Hg concentrates in the kidneys, where it is reabsorbed from the proximal tubules as Cys-S-Hg-S-Cys or in the basolateral membrane by organic anion transporters. Inorganic Hg cannot cross the blood-brain barrier or the placenta. Organic Hg is easily absorbed in the gastrointestinal tract (95%) and distributed throughout the body. Me-Hg binds to thiol-containing molecules (Me-Hg-Cys) to cross the blood-brain barrier. Mercury is excreted and accumulates in hair as Me-Hg, which is why this matrix is considered an index of exposure to the metal. Other forms of excretion are feces and urine [4, 28, 29].

Deposition and Effects of Mercury

In addition to the brain, mercury deposits in the thyroid, breasts, myocardium, muscles, adrenal, sweat, and salivary glands, liver, kidneys, skin, pancreas, enterocytes, lungs, testicles, and prostate. Mercury also has an affinity for binding sites on the surface of T cells and for sulfhydryl groups that influence T cell function. Specifically, Me-Hg easily deposits in the brain, liver, kidneys, placenta, and fetus, especially in the fetal brain, as well as in peripheral nerves and bone marrow. In the brain, Me-Hg demethylates to inorganic mercury and forms insoluble complexes with selenium that persist for years [4, 28, 29]. Additionally, mercury exposure can affect the immune system, causing allergies [30, 31].

Mercury and Poisoning

Two significant events in history have highlighted the dangers of mercury poisoning. The first occurred in Minamata, Japan, in the late 1950s, where an acetaldehyde factory contaminated Minamata Bay by releasing mercury-laden waste into Hyakken Port. In the water, Hg was transformed into Me-Hg and subsequently bioaccumulated by fish, which were the main food source for the local population. As a result, cats that ate the fish began to stagger and die. Subsequently, the local population was affected, particularly fetuses and developing children, with over two thousand people dying from this disaster and thousands more suffering irreversible damage. The second event occurred in Iraq in the 1970s when people consumed seed grains treated with a mercury-based fungicide [32, 33].

The damage caused by mercury exposure is known as Minamata disease, characterized by significant pathological changes in the central nervous system. Although mercury levels in the liver and kidneys are higher than in the central nervous system, the pathological changes are not as pronounced [28, 34]. Patients exhibit lesions in the cerebellar cortex, calcarine cortex, precentral gyrus, postcentral gyrus, and transverse temporal gyrus. Histopathologically, the brain shows a characteristic loss of neurons with gliosis in cortical layers II and III, regardless of severity. Characteristic cerebellar changes include the loss of granular cells and relatively well-preserved Purkinje cells [28, 35].

Mercury poisoning, like cadmium, can be acute or chronic, and its clinical manifestations will depend on the chemical form of the metal (see Table 6.2).

Clinical Manifestations of Elemental Mercury (Vapor) Poisoning

The primary target organ of mercury vapor is the brain; however, it is also associated with effects on peripheral nerves, renal function, immune function, endocrine and muscle function, and various types of dermatitis [29, 36].

Acute exposure to a large amount of mercury vapor induced erosive bronchitis, which can lead to respiratory failure. This is accompanied by central nervous system effects such as tremors or emotional changes (mood swings, irritability, nervousness, excessive shyness). In the case of chronic exposure, the symptoms are more subtle and non-specific: weakness, fatigue, anorexia, weight loss, and gastrointestinal discomfort. At higher exposures, fine tremors punctuated by a coarse tremor (myoclonus) occur; emotional changes, gingivitis, and excessive salivation, spasmodic postural tremors, psychotic behaviors, as well as immune dysfunction have also been described. These symptoms may regress with the cessation of exposure, but in many cases, they do not. Persistent neurological symptoms are common [29, 36].

Table 6.2 Type of poisoning and clinical outcomes

Type of poisoning	Metal/route	Inhalation	Oral	Dermal/ocular	Treatment
Acute	Cadmium	It can cause cough, dyspnea, headache, fever, and, if severe, chemical pneumonitis and non-cardiogenic pulmonary edema within 12–36 h after exposure	Colicky pain, diarrhea, local irritative processes (nausea, vomiting sometimes bloody). Within the first hour after consumption, metallic taste, myalgias, headaches, dysphagia, and salivation. Acute kidney failure. Altered liver function, metabolic acidosis, and coagulopathy	It can cause local irritation of the skin or eyes.	Symptomatic. The effectiveness of chelators such as EDTA, BAL, DPCN, DMPS, DMSA, MmDMSA, MiADMSA, MchDMSA, and DPCN is not fully proven
	Mercury	Mercury vapor induces erosive bronchitis and respiratory failure, tremors, or emotional changes	Elemental liquid mercury has not shown toxic effects. Ingestion of inorganic salts produces abdominal pain, bloody vomiting, and diarrhea with possible necrosis of the intestinal mucosa	Exposure to inorganic mercury salts: Skin rashes and dermatitis	Evaluate cardiovascular, respiratory, and airway status. Remove clothing if necessary. In case of skin exposure, wash with water and soap, and clean eyes with saline solution. Symptomatic patients require immediate treatment with chelating agents such as BAL, DPCN, DMPS, and DMSA. Remove the patient from the source of exposure
	Nickel	Asthma, bronchitis, rhinitis, sinusitis, respiratory tract and eye irritations, headaches, and fatigue have been reported	Nausea, vomiting, abdominal pain, diarrhea, headache, cough, shortness of breath, and dizziness	Redness, skin rashes, papules	The general condition of the patient should be evaluated considering possible exposure routes. A full physical examination, especially of the respiratory tract and skin, should be conducted management with chelating agents such as DMPS and DMSA and removal from exposure sources are necessary

Clinical Manifestations of Inorganic Mercury (Salts) Poisoning

Acute poisoning with mercury salts ($HgCl_2$) generally affects the gastrointestinal tract and kidneys. Extensive precipitation of enterocyte proteins occurs, with abdominal pain, vomiting, and bloody diarrhea with possible necrosis of the intestinal mucosa. This can lead to death from peritonitis or septic or hypovolemic shock. Patients who survive usually develop renal tubular necrosis with anuria. Chronic poisoning with mercury salts is rare and is generally associated with simultaneous occupational exposure to mercury vapor [29, 36].

Renal toxicity involves renal tubular necrosis or autoimmune glomerulonephritis, or both. Immune dysfunctions include hypersensitivity reactions to mercury exposure, such as asthma and dermatitis, various types of autoimmunity, and suppression of natural killer cells, as well as alteration of other lymphocyte subpopulations. Brain dysfunction is less evident than with other forms of mercury. Thyroid dysfunction appears to be associated with the inhibition of 5′ deiodinases, with a decrease in free T_3 and an increase in reverse T_3. Accumulation in the testes appears to inhibit spermatogenesis [29, 36].

Clinical Manifestations of Organic Mercury Poisoning

Methylmercury (Me-Hg) and ethylmercury (Et-Hg) produce similar signs and symptoms; however, most reports focus on Me-Hg. Symptoms are more related to the magnitude of methylmercury retention than the rate of deposition. Acute exposures tend to have a latency period of one or more weeks; once acquired, toxic doses are eliminated slowly in some cases [29, 36].

Massive prenatal poisoning can induce a form of cerebral palsy. Lower prenatal doses have been associated with delays in neurological development and cognitive deficits. Postnatal exposures generate a variety of symptoms ranging from paresthesias with minor exposures to ataxia, visual, auditory, and extrapyramidal deficits with moderate exposures, and clinic seizures in more severe exposures [29, 36].

Diagnosis of Mercury Poisoning

Diagnosing mercury concentrations in individuals is challenging. Commonly used modalities (levels in blood, urine, and/or hair) do not correlate with total body burden and offer little useful diagnostic information [29, 36–38].

In total blood, Hg concentration can be less than 10 μg/L, though 20 μg/L or less is considered normal. Blood Hg concentration can increase to 35 μg/L after prolonged exposure. Meanwhile, a urine Hg concentration >100 μg/L can trigger neurological symptoms in the patient, while levels of 800 μg/L can be fatal. Mercury concentrations in hair indicate prolonged exposure to the metal, specifically Me-Hg, with permissible levels being less than 1 mg/Kg [36].

Treatment of Mercury Poisoning

When mercury poisoning is suspected, an interview with the patient should be conducted to determine the source of exposure (environmental, occupational), followed by a physical examination. It is important to ascertain whether the exposure was chronic or acute and to eliminate the source. Cardiovascular, respiratory, and airway status should be evaluated. If necessary, clothing should be removed. In the case of skin exposure, it should be washed with soap and water. If the eyes were exposed, they should be rinsed with saline solution [36].

If a person has ingested or inhaled mercury, their respiratory status and oxygen saturation should be carefully monitored. If the patient exhibits symptoms such as difficulty breathing, a chest X-ray and arterial blood gas analysis should be performed, and preparations for intubation and artificial ventilation should be made. If intubation is necessary, removing liquid mercury through tracheal suction is useful to eliminate contamination [29, 36].

In cases where inorganic mercury compounds, such as liquid elemental mercury (Hg^0), have been ingested and there is no vomiting or aspiration, it is necessary to observe and monitor symptoms until the mercury is excreted from the body. At the same time, a kidney, ureter, and bladder X-ray can be used to track the movement of mercury through the gastrointestinal tract.

In the case of inorganic mercury compounds such as mercury chloride ($HgCl_2$), poisoning should be treated in the same manner as ingestion of corrosive substances due to the risk of damaging and perforating the mucosa of the gastrointestinal tract. In cases of acute gastrointestinal poisoning, symptomatic treatment is essential, such as evaluation of the airways, breathing, and cardiovascular status. Extensive intravenous therapy is necessary for a symptomatic patient. Additionally, the condition of the laryngopharynx and gastrointestinal tract should be assessed on an empty stomach. If the examined areas are intact, gastric lavage with activated charcoal is performed. Finally, blood dialysis is an essential intervention in the treatment of renal failure caused by inorganic mercury poisoning.

Symptomatic patients with mercury poisoning require immediate treatment with chelating agents. However, the use of this therapy should be evaluated according to the patient's condition. As with cadmium poisoning, BAL, DPCN, DMPS, and DMSA are commonly used for acute Hg^0 poisoning. Among these chelators, BAL is contraindicated as a treatment for organic mercury poisoning. DPCN increases the excretion of lead and mercury (elemental and inorganic) through the urine. For mercury poisoning, adults are treated with 250 mg of DPCN orally four times a day for 1 or 2 weeks, while children receive 20–30 mg/kg per day divided into four doses (maximum 250 mg/dose). Adverse effects of the agent include leukopenia, thrombocytopenia, aplastic anemia, proteinuria, hematuria, and nephrotic syndrome. DMSA has been frequently used to replace DPCN, given its great metal-carrying capacity and fewer side effects. BAL is administered only by intramuscular injection, which causes pain. This agent has a narrow therapeutic window and a risk of allergic reaction. Recent substitutes for BAL include DMSA and DMPS.

DMSA has a half-life of about 3 h, which is prolonged in children and people poisoned by mercury. When administered orally, its absorption rate is around 20%. This agent increases urinary excretion of methylmercury and inorganic mercury. In animal tests, it has been reported to be effective in promoting the excretion of methylmercury from the brain, so it is widely used to treat severe cases of Me-Hg poisoning. DMSA can be taken orally to minimize its adverse effects; however, patients may rarely experience mucocutaneous rash and toxic epidermal necrolysis, which resolve once the drug administration is discontinued.

The absorption rate of DMPS is around 39% when taken orally, although due to its stability, it is frequently administered intravenously. Like DMSA, DMPS induces the excretion of Me-Hg and inorganic mercury in the urine; however, it is not effective for eliminating methylmercury through the kidneys to remove methylmercury from the brain.

Mercury and Allergies

As previously described, mercury can be found in three forms in the environment: elemental mercury (Hg°), inorganic mercury (Hg^{+} and Hg^{2+}), and organic mercury (methyl, ethyl, and phenyl). This metal has been characterized for its use in health and aesthetic purposes. Mercury is a metal known in the contexts of allergy, hypersensitivity, and even autoimmunity. For sensitization to this metal to occur, there must have been exposure to low concentrations of metal, which differ from intoxication because their levels in blood, urine, or hair are normal. Such exposures can vary due to the forms of mercury, and thus, we commonly find ethyl mercury in dental amalgam used for restoration of dental pieces, in the thimerosal preservative found in vaccines like influenza, and in makeup; methylmercury in fish consumption; elemental mercury in thermometers, barometers, and other electrical devices we frequently use; and inorganic mercury, which is widely used in the cosmetology area, soap and cream making. Therefore, it is very easy to be exposed to mercury and develop sensitization processes.

When a person is already sensitized and comes into contact with the metal that triggers a type IV hypersensitivity allergic reaction, it can be a delayed reaction; hence, it may take days to develop and is not mediated by antibodies but by activated CD8 cells. The metal in its elemental state does not produce a hypersensitive reaction; it must undergo an ionization process that facilitates its contact with body fluids, causing the metal to bind to proteins. Subsequently, the immune system of sensitized people recognizes these bonds as foreign bodies and reacts, causing chronic inflammation that can be associated with various chronic clinical manifestations.

Clinical Manifestations of Mercury Allergy

Like other metals, mercury has been associated with the appearance of allergic dermatitis syndromes (baboon syndrome), which can be triggered by the use of amalgams or by inhalation of the metal. Additionally, it is the most common symptom in patients exposed to mercury, characterized by erythema with well-defined borders in the gluteal/perianal region and/or V-shaped erythema in the inguinal/perigenital area, with symmetry of the affected areas and absence of systemic symptoms and signs [40]. Other conditions described include contact dermatitis, presenting with eczema, itching, inflammation, redness, and heat, as well as stomatitis and gingivitis. There is an association with the development of asthma, uncertain chronic fatigue, neuropathic pain, fibromyalgia, musculoskeletal pain, and remodeling of oral tissue, which can lead to oral lichen planus [41–44]. Patients allergic to orthopedic prostheses and those experiencing facial dermatitis from makeup containing mercury derivatives have also been affected [39, 45].

Diagnosis and Treatment of Mercury-Induced Allergy

To diagnose mercury allergy, there are several methods, such as the MELISA test (Memory Lymphocyte Immunostimulation Assay), which assesses cellular activity compared to the same cells not exposed to any metal and measures the level of allergy through microscopic observation, comparing lymphocyte proliferation before and after exposure to the metal in question. Another method is the patch test or skin test, which is based on exposure to the metal and waiting for a dermal allergic reaction. Measuring metal levels in blood, urine, or hair is not recommended because concentrations in blood are normal and do not identify allergy. If there is an elevation in blood, the patient would be experiencing intoxication [44, 46].

Nickel

Nickel (Ni) is a metal first isolated in 1751 by Swedish scientist Axel Fredrik Cronstedt. It is the fifth most common chemical element on Earth, found in the crust, core, and mantle, and the 22nd most common element on Earth (0.008% of the Earth's crust and 0.01% of igneous rocks), and the seventh among transition elements. There are 24 known isotopes of nickel, five of which are natural [47]. It has an atomic number of 28, an atomic weight of 58.7, and the symbol Ni, located in group 10 of the periodic table among the transition elements, and classified as a ferrous metal as it belongs to the Iron triad: Iron, Nickel, and Cobalt [48]. It has very useful physical and chemical properties, such as malleability, good thermal conductivity, high ductility, resistance to atmospheric agents, ferromagnetism, moderate hardness, and poor electrical conductivity, making it one of the most commercialized and used metals in the world [47, 48].

It is a hard, white-silver metal that can be mixed with other metals, such as iron, copper, chromium, and zinc to form alloys. These alloys are used to make coins, jewelry, metal tools, utensils, keys, and medical devices, especially those for orthopedic use, orthodontics, and cardiovascular prostheses. It is also found in some foods such as chocolate, salmon, peanuts, and legumes. Additionally, it can combine with other elements like chlorine, sulfur, and oxygen to form nickel compounds with different oxidation states, such as nickel oxide, nickel hydroxide, nickel chloride, and nickel sulfate, which are used for ceramic coloring, making catalysts, and batteries. Normally, we can find it in soils, volcanic emissions, meteorites, and ocean floors. This chemical element and its derivatives have no characteristic odor or taste. Most nickel is used to make stainless steel, making it a very abundant natural element [49].

Nickel is released into the atmosphere by industries that manufacture nickel, its alloys, and compounds. Its release can be through air or industrial wastewater. When the particles of the element are in the air, they adhere to small dust particles that settle on the ground or are removed by rain and/or snow. However, when nickel is released into industrial wastewater, it ends up in sediment, where it strongly adheres to particles containing iron or manganese [47]. It is also emitted into the atmosphere by plants that burn oil or coal and by incineration of garbage.

There are different types of nickel exposure, which can occur through four routes: percutaneous absorption, ingestion, and inhalation. The relevant route is through the skin, especially after repeated cutaneous exposures, such as skin contact with soil, bath or shower water, and metals containing nickel, as well as touching coins or jewelry. However, there are other common sources of exposure, such as inhalation of air contaminated with nickel or tobacco in the form of nickel carbonyl, where concentrations range from 1.1 to 3.1 μg, and 10% to 20% of inhaled nickel is in the gas phase. Oral ingestion of contaminated food or liquids produces negative gastrointestinal effects. It has been reported that the source of exposure with the highest amount of nickel is among workers in industries that process or use nickel, who can be exposed to very high amounts of this metal, which can cause systemic inflammatory damage, cancer, and allergic reactions [49].

Nickel and Poisoning

Given the abundance of this chemical element on Earth, humans are constantly exposed to nickel, making it a significant public health issue. It is a hemotoxic, immunotoxic, neurotoxic, genotoxic, nephrotoxic, and hepatotoxic chemical agent. It can cause toxicities with side effects on the male and female reproductive systems, leading to infertility at concentrations of 10–20 mg/kg. Additionally, cases of pulmonary toxicity with carcinogenic potential have been reported [48].

The size of its particles is important to determine where deposits would be in the body. Water-soluble nickel compounds are absorbed through the lungs by diffusion, while water-insoluble compounds enter the respiratory system by phagocytosis and remain in the lungs for a longer time. Nevertheless, the main target organ for its deposition is the kidney, with other deposition sites including the brain and the pancreas. The transport of this metal in the body occurs through the binding of the metal ion with specific serum proteins such as albumin, L-histidine, and α-2 macroglobulin. Its metabolism involves the exchange of nickel ions with other ionic sources. It is known that nickel interferes with the physiological processes of multiple metals, which explains the physiological manifestation of its toxicity. The excretion pathways are urine and/or feces, depending on the route of exposure and the ionic state of the exposure [50, 51].

Regardless of occupational or non-occupational exposure, the exposed person will develop a reaction or intoxication that will manifest as a symptom or clinical sign. In the case of intoxication, the type of exposure should be identified—whether it was inhaled as nickel carbonyl or ingested accidentally, such as water used in washing and purifying metals. Normally, gastrointestinal tract symptoms take hours or 2 days to disappear. When inhaled, acute nickel toxicity is more frequently observed, producing renal injury, frank hematuria, frontal headache, nausea, vomiting, chest pain, and 40% of patients present respiratory symptoms within the first hour after exposure. Chronic exposure can be observed after several hours, or even several days, depending on the intensity of the exposure. Symptoms are associated with visceral damage, producing hepatic toxicities, myocarditis, hypothermia, interstitial pneumonia, rhinitis, renal tubular degeneration, and incidence of reproductive and developmental toxicity, even leading to death due to complications from interstitial pneumonia or cerebral edema [47].

The International Agency for Research on Cancer and the U.S. Department of Health and Human Services have classified insoluble nickel compounds as one of the most potent human carcinogens. The critical processes involved in carcinogenic action include oxidative stress, genomic DNA damage, epigenetic changes, and altered regulation of gene expression through the activation of transcription factors such as NF-Kβ, HIF-1, ATF-1, p53, and Rb protein. These factors are stimulated in nickel-modified cells, contributing to cell cycle deregulation, cell proliferation, increased tumor growth, and allergic effects that eventually lead to cancer, especially those affecting the lungs and paranasal sinuses [50, 51].

Clinical Manifestations of Nickel Poisoning

Nickel toxicity depends on the route of exposure, amount, and concentration. In this regard, intoxication can be acute or chronic, depending on the route of exposure (Table 6.1). In one-day-old intoxications, values of 1.63 g/L were found, with different symptoms such as nausea, vomiting, abdominal pain, diarrhea, headache, cough, shortness of breath, and dizziness, which lasted for a maximum of two days, accompanied by increased urinary albumin, without showing major tubular damage. From 10 days to 110 days, it was found that at concentrations of 0.07–1.1 mg Ni/m^3, there was an increase in irritations in the respiratory tract and eyes, headaches, and fatigue. There was an increase in urinary levels of total protein, β2-microglobulin, retinal-binding protein, and N-acetyl-β-D-glucosaminidase (NAG). Despite possible tubular dysfunction, no damage to glomerular function was reported by the markers. After more than 100 days, asthma, bronchitis, rhinitis, sinusitis, and pneumoconiosis have been reported [47, 51]. On the skin, it has been described that it produces contact dermatitis, developing complications such as skin redness, rashes, pustules, and ulcers [50, 52]. Other symptoms it can cause include hearing loss, damage to the retina or optic nerve, altered estrogen levels, chromosome abnormalities, or chronic inflammation [49].

Diagnosis of Nickel Poisoning

A thorough anamnesis is required for its diagnosis because, like all metal intoxications, its symptoms are very non-specific, making diagnosis difficult without the history of metal exposure. Table 6.1 shows the clinical manifestations according to the route of exposure. Initially, control blood tests, biochemistry, and blood gases are requested in cases where the exposure route was inhalation, as nickel carbonyl causes early hypoxia. The measurement of nickel levels in blood and urine is the standard test to assess toxicity levels, which will depend on the amount of nickel deposited and the duration of exposure. An EKG is also ordered in cases of myocarditis, where QT prolongation and ST-T changes can be observed. Chest X-rays show non-specific infiltrates that develop as pneumonitis progresses [49].

Treatment of Nickel Poisoning

Emergency and Support Measures [50]

Initially, exposure to the toxicant should be interrupted, and the source of exposure should be eliminated as quickly as possible, starting with decontamination and supportive medical management.

Inhalation: Respiratory symptoms should be managed by administering O_2 to manage hypoxia, bronchodilators, and corticosteroids to treat associated bronchospasm and mechanical ventilation in severe cases.

Percutaneous Absorption: If exposure was cutaneous, clothes should be removed, and skin decontamination should be performed to interrupt exposure and absorption through the skin.

Ingestion: Manage fluid loss due to gastroenteritis with IV crystalloid fluids and perform gastric lavage following considerable ingestion of the metal.

Drugs and Specific Antidotes

The pharmacological management of nickel intoxications is primarily through chelation treatments. Sodium diethyldithiocarbamate (Dithiocarb) has been shown to be a specific antidote for inhalation of nickel carbonyl; tetraethylthiuram (Antabuse) is effective to a lesser extent; D-penicillamine and dimercaprol (BAL) have limited therapeutic value. For the treatment of nickel eczema and dermatitis, a favorable response was obtained by subjecting patients to a low-nickel diet along with the oral administration of Dithiocarb or Antabuse. Specific treatments for nickel-induced cancer have not yet been reported, and the creation of new chelators that prevent the phases of the carcinogenic process is awaited [53].

Nickel and Allergies

Nickel is the metal with the highest incidence of contact hypersensitivity and the most frequent positive allergen in patients with patch tests for suspected ACD. For this reason, in 2008, it was named the "Contact Allergen of the Year" by the American Contact Dermatitis Society (ACDS) [54].

It is a relevant allergen with many exposure sources. Nickel sensitization can occur at any age, but once developed, it lasts a lifetime, reducing the quality of life. It has been observed that sensitization is more frequent in women than men, possibly due to constant use of items such as jewelry and the manufacturing process. Sensitization has been reported in musicians, especially violinists, cellists, guitarists, flutists, and trumpeters, as well as in the use of prosthetics, surgical instruments, and cell phones. However, epidemiological studies have shown a higher incidence of nickel sensitization in atopic individuals [55].

Nickel sensitization is a type IV hypersensitivity, associated with the metal and its water-soluble alloys, such as nickel chloride ($NiCl_2$) and nickel sulfate ($NiSO_4$). This metal forms stable complexes with soluble skin proteins, replacing other ions and altering protein conformation, making them antigenically active, provoking an inflammatory response in the skin known as a delayed-type hypersensitivity (DTH) reaction [55].

Clinical Manifestations of Nickel Allergy

The typical clinical presentation is allergic contact dermatitis (ACD), which appears as eczematous dermatitis localized at sites of persistent contact with metal-containing objects. Systemic exposure to metals (ingestion, inhalation, or infusion) in sensitized patients can cause generalized dermatitis, called systemic contact dermatitis, accompanied by erythematous, papular, edematous, and vesicular lesions. Chronic episodes can show lichenified lesions. The most common sites of appearance are the hands, fingers, ears, periumbilical region, and thoracoabdominal area. Table 6.2 shows other associated clinical manifestations [54, 56]. Other non-eczematous reactions include erythema multiforme-like lesions, lichenoid reactions with cutaneous, and especially oral mucosal involvement. Other clinical patterns include granuloma annulare-like reactions, vitiligo-like lesions, lymphomatoid contact dermatitis, sycosis-like dermatitis of the beard, dyshidrosiform pemphigoid, and vasculitis [54, 57, 58].

Diagnosis of Nickel Allergy

Although clinical evaluation and thorough anamnesis are essential for diagnosis, the patch test is the gold standard for diagnosing ACD. The patch test reading is done 48, 72, or 96 h after applying the metal to the skin. It is considered positive when the evaluation shows the presence of erythematous, infiltrative, papular, and vesicular lesions according to ICDRG criteria. Irritant pustular reactions can also be observed due to different nickel alloys with other metals. The oral provocation test, where a certain amount of metal is administered to evaluate the flare reaction, defined as the reactivation or activation of previous patch test sites due to systemic exposure to an allergen, is also used [59].

Treatment of Nickel Allergy

The best solution for sensitization to this allergen is avoidance. Therefore, avoiding contact with nickel is the best way to treat and prevent ACD induced by this metal. It is recommended not to use any material that may contain the metal or, alternatively, use materials made from other chemical elements. If one must work exclusively with nickel, a physical barrier should be created to avoid direct contact (safety protection elements). Reducing high-nickel diets and properly caring for kitchen utensils are also advised. In cases of acute allergic contact dermatitis, in addition to measures to avoid contact with the metal, topical or systemic corticosteroids will be prescribed. Disulfiram, which acts as a nickel chelating agent, has also been reported in the treatment of nickel dermatitis. As a precautionary method, the European Community Regulation on chemicals and their safe use (Registration, Evaluation, Authorization of Chemicals) prohibits the release of more than 0.5 μg of nickel/cm^2/week from metallic products. However, it remains the main allergen triggering ACD [54, 55].

Conclusion

In recent years, it has been observed that heavy metals are responsible for toxicological and allergic processes that can lead to the development of diseases and even death. It is essential to clearly understand the pathophysiological and symptomatic differences by which metals can be associated with intoxication and allergies or hypersensitivity reactions. Although intoxications are known to be the main cause of diseases associated with metal exposure, allergies have gained prominence in this field, making it necessary to be prepared with the necessary measures for their management. The scientific community is invited to establish management protocols for both cases to optimize patient management and response time, with clear objectives and ensuring the patient's life is safeguarded.

Glossary

Glossary of Acronyms

AAAAI American Academy of Allergy, Asthma, and Immunology
ADH Alcohol Dehydrogenase
ALDH Aldehyde Dehydrogenase
CMA Cow's Milk Allergy
CoMiSS Cow's Milk-related Symptom Score
DSM-V Diagnostic and Statistical Manual of Mental Disorders, Fifth Edition
EAACI European Academy of Allergy and Clinical Immunology
EHF Extensively Hydrolyzed Formula
GI Gastrointestinal
IgE Immunoglobulin E
LI Lactose Intolerance
NAD Nicotinamide Adenine Dinucleotide
NAD+ Nicotinamide Adenine Dinucleotide (oxidized form)
NADH Nicotinamide Adenine Dinucleotide (reduced form)
REM Rapid Eye Movement
SGLT-1 Sodium/Glucose Cotransporter 1
SPT Skin Prick Test
Th2 T-helper 2 cells
TNF-α Tumor Necrosis Factor-alpha
WHO World Health Organization

Glossary of Terms

Acute Intoxication Rapid onset of symptoms following exposure to a toxic substance.

Atopic Dermatitis A type of inflammation of the skin (eczema), often associated with allergies.

BAL (British Anti-Lewisite) A chelating agent used in the treatment of heavy metal poisoning.

Cadmium (Cd) A heavy metal with no biological function in humans, often associated with industrial pollution.

Chelation Therapy Treatment that involves the administration of chelating agents to remove heavy metals from the body.

Chronic Exposure Prolonged exposure to a toxic substance, often leading to long-term health effects.

Contact Dermatitis Inflammation of the skin caused by contact with certain substances.

Dermal Absorption The process by which a substance passes through the skin and into the body.

DMPS (2,3-Dimercapto-1-propanesulfonic acid) A chelating agent used to treat heavy metal poisoning.

DMSA (2,3-Dimercaptosuccinic acid) A chelating agent used to treat heavy metal poisoning.

Elemental Mercury (Hg0) The pure form of mercury, which is liquid at room temperature and highly toxic.

IgE (Immunoglobulin E) An antibody associated with allergic reactions.

Inhalation Exposure The intake of substances through breathing.

Mercury (Hg) A highly toxic heavy metal that exists in elemental, inorganic, and organic forms.

Metallothioneins Proteins that bind heavy metals and aid in their detoxification.

Methylmercury (Me-Hg) A highly toxic form of mercury found in certain fish and seafood.

Nickel (Ni) A heavy metal commonly associated with allergic reactions and contact dermatitis.

Non-Essential Heavy Metals Metals that have no beneficial role in biological systems and are toxic even at low concentrations.

Patch Test A diagnostic tool used to identify allergic reactions to various substances.

Thimerosal An organic mercury compound used as a preservative in vaccines and other products.

References

1. Rehman K, Fatima F, Waheed I, Akash MSH. Prevalence of exposure of heavy metals and their impact on health consequences. J Cell Biochem [Internet]. 2018 [cited 2022 Sep 5];119(1):157–84. Available from: https://pubmed.ncbi.nlm.nih.gov/28643849/.
2. Izah SC, Inyang IR, Angaye TCN, Okowa IP. A review of heavy metal concentration and potential health implications of beverages consumed in Nigeria. Toxics [Internet]. 2017 [cited 2022 Sep 5];5(1). Available from: https://pmc.ncbi.nlm.nih.gov/articles/PMC5606672/.
3. Witkowska D, Słowik J, Chilicka K. Heavy metals and human health: possible exposure pathways and the competition for protein binding sites. Molecules [Internet]. 2021 [cited 2022 Sep 5];26(19). Available from: https://pmc.ncbi.nlm.nih.gov/articles/PMC8511997/.
4. Hejna M, Gottardo D, Baldi A, Dell'Orto V, Cheli F, Zaninelli M, et al. Review: nutritional ecology of heavy metals. Animal. 2018;12(10):2156–70.
5. Hsieh CY, Jung CR, Lin CY, Hwang BF. Combined exposure to heavy metals in PM2.5 and pediatric asthma. J Allergy Clin Immunol. 2021;147(6):2171–2180.e13.
6. Tsai TL, Wang SL, Hsieh CJ, Wen HJ, Kuo CC, Liu HJ, et al. Association between prenatal exposure to metals and atopic dermatitis among children aged 4 years in Taiwan. JAMA Netw Open [Internet]. 2021 [cited 2022 Sep 3];4(10). Available from: https://pubmed.ncbi.nlm.nih.gov/34705012/.
7. Granum B, Oftedal B, Agier L, Siroux V, Bird P, Casas M, et al. Multiple environmental exposures in early-life and allergy-related outcomes in childhood. Environ Int. 2020;144:106038.
8. Satarug S. Dietary cadmium intake and its effects on kidneys. Toxics [Internet]. 2018 [cited 2022 Aug 30];6(1). Available from: https://pmc.ncbi.nlm.nih.gov/articles/PMC5874788/.
9. Genchi G, Sinicropi MS, Lauria G, Carocci A, Catalano A. The effects of cadmium toxicity. Int J Environ Res Public Health [Internet]. 2020 [cited 2022 Aug 30];17(11). Available from: https://pmc.ncbi.nlm.nih.gov/articles/PMC7312803/.
10. Lane EA, Canty MJ, More SJ. Cadmium exposure and consequence for the health and productivity of farmed ruminants. Res Vet Sci. 2015;101:132–9.
11. Rahimzadeh MR, Rahimzadeh MR, Kazemi S, Moghadamnia AA. Cadmium toxicity and treatment: an update. Caspian J Intern Med [Internet]. 2017 [cited 2022 Aug 30];8(3):135. Available from: https://pmc.ncbi.nlm.nih.gov/articles/PMC5596182/.
12. Jacobo-Estrada T, Cardenas-Gonzalez M, Santoyo-Sánchez MP, Thevenod F, Barbier O. Intrauterine exposure to cadmium reduces HIF-1 DNA-binding ability in rat fetal kidneys. Toxics [Internet]. 2018 [cited 2022 Sep 3];6(3). Available from: https://pmc.ncbi.nlm.nih.gov/articles/PMC6161213/.
13. Lu Y, Wu J, Gu W, Huang Z, Shu Z, Huang M, et al. Single-cell transcriptomics uncovers phenotypic alterations in the monocytes in a Chinese population with chronic cadmium exposure. Ecotoxicol Environ Saf. 2021;211:111881.
14. Schaefer HR, Flannery BM, Crosby L, Jones-Dominic OE, Punzalan C, Middleton K. A systematic review of adverse health effects associated with oral cadmium exposure. Regul Toxicol Pharmacol [Internet]. 2022 [cited 2022 Aug 30];134:105243. Available from: https://linkinghub.elsevier.com/retrieve/pii/S0273230022001301.
15. Wang P, Chen H, Kopittke PM, Zhao FJ. Cadmium contamination in agricultural soils of China and the impact on food safety. Environ Pollut. 2019;249:1038–48.
16. Ministerio de Salud. Dirección General de Salud de las Personas. Guia de Práctica Clínica para el Diagnóstico y Tratamiento de la Intoxicación por Cadmio [Internet]. Lima; 2015 pp. 3–25. Available from: http://www.minsa.gob.pe.
17. Zahedi A, Hassanvand MS, Jaafarzadeh N, Ghadiri A, Shamsipour M, Dehcheshmeh MG. Effect of ambient air PM2.5-bound heavy metals on blood metal(loid)s and children's asthma and allergy pro-inflammatory (IgE, IL-4 and IL-13) biomarkers. J Trace Elem Med Biol. 2021;(68):126826.

18. Mirkov I, Popov Aleksandrov A, Ninkov M, Tucovic D, Kulas J, Zeljkovic M, et al. Immunotoxicology of cadmium: cells of the immune system as targets and effectors of cadmium toxicity. Food Chem Toxicol. 2021;149:112026.
19. Zeng X, Xu X, Zheng X, Reponen T, Chen A, Huo X. Heavy metals in PM2.5 and in blood, and children's respiratory symptoms and asthma from an e-waste recycling area. Environ Pollut [Internet]. 2016 [cited 2022 Sep 3];210:346–53. Available from: https://pubmed.ncbi.nlm.nih.gov/26803791/.
20. Yang G, Sun T, Han YY, Rosser F, Forno E, Chen W, et al. Serum cadmium and lead, current wheeze, and lung function in a Nationwide study of adults in the United States. J Allergy Clin Immunol Pract. 2019;7(8):2653–2660.e3.
21. Kim JH, Jeong KS, Ha EH, Park H, Ha M, Hong YC, et al. Association between prenatal exposure to cadmium and atopic dermatitis in infancy. J Korean Med Sci [Internet]. 2013 [cited 2022 Sep 3];28(4):516. Available from: https://pmc.ncbi.nlm.nih.gov/articles/PMC3617302/.
22. Pesce G, Sesé L, Calciano L, Travert B, Dessimond B, Maesano CN, et al. Foetal exposure to heavy metals and risk of atopic diseases in early childhood. Pediatr Allergy Immunol [Internet]. 2021 Feb 1 [cited 2022 Sep 3];32(2):242–50. Available from: https://pubmed.ncbi.nlm.nih.gov/33091176/
23. Lin H, Ascher DB, Myung Y, Lamborg CH, Hallam SJ, Gionfriddo CM, et al. Mercury methylation by metabolically versatile and cosmopolitan marine bacteria. ISME J [Internet]. 2021 [cited 2022 Sep 10];15(6):1810–25. Available from: https://pubmed.ncbi.nlm.nih.gov/33504941/
24. Yang L, Zhang Y, Wang F, Luo Z, Guo S, Strähle U. Toxicity of mercury: Molecular evidence. Chemosphere [Internet]. 2020 [cited 2022 Sep 7];245. Available from: https://pubmed.ncbi.nlm.nih.gov/31881386/.
25. Santos-Sacramento L, Arrifano GP, Lopes-Araújo A, Augusto-Oliveira M, Albuquerque-Santos R, Takeda PY, et al. Human neurotoxicity of mercury in the Amazon: a scoping review with insights and critical considerations. Ecotoxicol Environ Saf. 2021;208:111686.
26. Ijaz MU, Majeed SA, Asharaf A, Ali T, Al-Ghanim KA, Asad F, et al. Toxicological effects of thimerosal on rat kidney: a histological and biochemical study. Braz J Biol [Internet]. 2021 [cited 2022 Sep 10];83. Available from: https://pubmed.ncbi.nlm.nih.gov/34468508/.
27. Lavoie RA, Bouffard A, Maranger R, Amyot M. Mercury transport and human exposure from global marine fisheries. Sci Rep [Internet]. 2018 Dec 1 [cited 2022 Sep 10];8(1). Available from: https://pubmed.ncbi.nlm.nih.gov/29712952/.
28. Balali-Mood M, Naseri K, Tahergorabi Z, Khazdair MR, Sadeghi M. Toxic mechanisms of five heavy metals: mercury, lead, chromium, cadmium, and arsenic. Front Pharmacol [Internet]. 2021 [cited 2022 Sep 10];12. Available from: https://pmc.ncbi.nlm.nih.gov/articles/PMC8078867/.
29. Bernhoft RA. Mercury toxicity and treatment: a review of the literature. J Environ Public Health [Internet]. 2012 [cited 2022 Sep 7];2012. Available from: https://pmc.ncbi.nlm.nih.gov/articles/PMC3253456/.
30. Pollard KM, Cauvi DM, Toomey CB, Hultman P, Kono DH. Mercury-induced inflammation and autoimmunity. Biochim Biophys Acta Gen Subj [Internet]. 2019 [cited 2022 Sep 10];1863(12):129299. Available from: https://pmc.ncbi.nlm.nih.gov/articles/PMC6689266/.
31. Peng B, Che D, Hao Y, Zheng Y, Liu R, Qian Y, et al. Thimerosal induces skin pseudo-allergic reaction via mas-related G-protein coupled receptor B2. J Dermatol Sci [Internet]. 2019 [cited 2022 Sep 10];95(3):99–106. Available from: https://pubmed.ncbi.nlm.nih.gov/31558225/
32. Skerfving SB, Copplestone JF. Poisoning caused by the consumption of organomercury-dressed seed in Iraq. Bull World Health Organ [Internet] 1976 [cited 2022 Sep 10];54(1):101. Available from: https://pmc.ncbi.nlm.nih.gov/articles/PMC2366450/.
33. Yoshino K, Mori K, Kanaya G, Kojima S, Henmi Y, Matsuyama A, et al. Food sources are more important than biomagnification on mercury bioaccumulation in marine fishes. Environ Pollut [Internet]. 2020 Jul 1 [cited 2022 Sep 10];262. Available from: https://pubmed.ncbi.nlm.nih.gov/32146359/

34. Ganguly J, Kulshreshtha D, Jog M. Mercury and movement disorders: the toxic legacy continues. Can J Neurol Sci [Internet]. 2022 [cited 2022 Sep 10];49(4):493–501. Available from: https://pubmed.ncbi.nlm.nih.gov/34346303/
35. Marumoto M, Sakamoto M, Marumoto K, Tsuruta S, Komohara Y. Mercury and Selenium Localization in the Cerebrum, Cerebellum, Liver, and Kidney of a Minamata Disease Case. Acta Histochem Cytochem [Internet]. 2020 Dec 12 [cited 2022 Sep 10];53(6):147. Available from: https://pmc.ncbi.nlm.nih.gov/articles/PMC7785461/.
36. Ye BJ, Kim BG, Jeon MJ, Kim SY, Kim HC, Jang TW, et al. Evaluation of mercury exposure level, clinical diagnosis and treatment for mercury intoxication. Ann Occup Environ Med [Internet]. 2016 [cited 2022 Sep 10];28(1). Available from: https://pmc.ncbi.nlm.nih.gov/articles/PMC4724159/.
37. Amadi CN, Offor SJ, Frazzoli C, Orisakwe OE. Natural antidotes and management of metal toxicity. Environ Sci Pollut Res Int [Internet]. 2019 [cited 2022 Sep 10];26(18):18032–52. Available from: https://pubmed.ncbi.nlm.nih.gov/31079302/.
38. Kim JJ, Kim YS, Kumar V. Heavy metal toxicity: an update of chelating therapeutic strategies. J Trace Elem Med Biol [Internet]. 2019 [cited 2022 Sep 10];54:226–31. Available from: https://pubmed.ncbi.nlm.nih.gov/31109617/.
39. Haddad SF, Helm MM, Meath B, Adams C, Packianathan N, Uhl R. Exploring the incidence, implications, and relevance of metal allergy to Orthopaedic surgeons. J Am Acad Orthop Surg Glob Res Rev. 2019;3(4)
40. Tan MG, Pratt MD, Burns BF, Glassman SJ. Baboon syndrome from mercury showing leukocytoclastic vasculitis on biopsy. Vol. 83, contact dermatitis. Blackwell Publishing Ltd; 2020. p. 415–7.
41. Kim KN, Bae S, Park HY, Kwon HJ, Hong YC. Low-level mercury exposure and risk of asthma in school-age children. Epidemiology. 2015;26(5):733–9.
42. Stejskal VDM, Forsbeck M, Cederbrant KE, Asteman O. Mercury-specific lymphocytes: an indication of mercury allergy in man. J Clin Immunol. 1996;16:31.
43. 1995. Oral lichenoid lesions, mercury hypersensitivity an combined hypersensitivity to mercury and other metals.
44. Contact_allergies_to_dental_materials.
45. Pigatto PD, Guzzi G. Allergy to gold: the two faces of mercury. Vol. 29, Annals of dermatology. Korean Dermatological Association; 2017. p. 105–6.
46. Mercury-methylmercury-allergy.
47. Das KK, Reddy RC, Bagoji IB, Das S, Bagali S, Mullur L, et al. Primary concept of nickel toxicity—an overview. J Basic Clin Physiol Pharmacol De Gruyter 30 2019. p. 141–152.
48. Rizvi A, Parveen S, Khan S, Naseem I. Nickel toxicology with reference to male molecular reproductive physiology. In: Reproductive biology, vol. 20. Elsevier Sp. z o.o; 2020. p. 3–8.
49. Genchi G, Carocci A, Lauria G, Sinicropi MS, Catalano A. Nickel: human health and environmental toxicology. Int J Environ Res Public Health MDPI AG; 17, 2020.
50. Lluis A. Toxicologia do Níquel Toxicology of Nickel.
51. Schreiver I, Hesse B, Seim C, Castillo-Michel H, Anklamm L, Villanova J, et al. Distribution of nickel and chromium containing particles from tattoo needle wear in humans and its possible impact on allergic reactions. Part Fibre Toxicol. 2019;16(1):33.
52. Ahlström MG, Midander K, Menné T, Lidén C, Johansen JD, Julander A, et al. Nickel deposition and penetration into the stratum corneum after short metallic nickel contact: an experimental study. Contact Derm. 2019;80(2):86–93.
53. Andersen O, Aaseth J. A review of pitfalls and progress in chelation treatment of metal poisonings. J Trace Elements Med Biol Elsevier GmbH. 2016;38:74–80.
54. Silverberg NB, Pelletier JL, Jacob SE, Schneider LC, Cohen B, Horii KA, et al. Nickel allergic contact dermatitis: identification, treatment, and prevention. Pediatrics. 2020;145(5)
55. Tramontana M, Bianchi L, Hansel K, Agostinelli D, Stingeni L. Nickel allergy: epidemiology, pathomechanism, clinical patterns, treatment and prevention programs. Endocr Metab Immune Disord Drug Targets. 2020;20(7):992–1002.

56. Ricciardi L, Minciullo PL, Saitta S. Systemic nickel allergy syndrome: tips and tricks on how to be suspected and treated [Internet]. J Biol Regul Homeost Agents. 2019. Available from: https://www.researchgate.net/publication/334883984.
57. Anna BM, Grazyna A, Wojciech D, Aleksander O, Anna B, Andrzej K, et al. Nickel allergy and relationship with Staphylococcus aureus in atopic dermatitis. J Trace Elem Med Biol. 2016;33:1–7.
58. Borghi A, Corazza M, Maietti E, Patruno C, Napolitano M, Schena D, et al. Eyelid dermatitis and contact sensitization to nickel: results from an Italian multi-centric observational study. Endocr Metab Immune Disord Drug Targets. 2019;19(1):38–45.
59. Ahlström MG, Thyssen JP, Wennervaldt M, Menné T, Johansen JD. Nickel allergy and allergic contact dermatitis: a clinical review of immunology, epidemiology, exposure, and treatment, vol. 81. Contact Dermatitis. Blackwell Publishing Ltd; 2019. p. 227–41.

Further Readings

Shin J, Kim BM, Ha M, Park HS, Hong YC, Kim Y, et al. The association between mercury exposure and atopic dermatitis in early childhood: a mothers and children's environmental health study. Epidemiology. 2019;30:S3–8.

Stejskal V. Allergy and autoimmunity caused by metals: a unifying concept. In: Vaccines and autoimmunity. Wiley Blackwell; 2014. p. 57–63.

Cederbrant K, Hultman P. Characterization of mercuric mercury (Hg 21)-induced lymphoblasts from patients with mercury allergy and from healthy subjects. Clin Exp Immunol. 2000;121(1):23–30. https://doi.org/10.1046/j.1365-2249.2000.01268.x. PMID: 10886235; PMCID: PMC1905683.

Chapter 7
Toxicity and Allergies to Medications

Neyder Contreras-Puentes, Maryarena Castro-Leones, Brandon Gutiérrez-Tovar, and Jorge Mendoza-Galiz

Introduction

Medications are agents intended for the prevention and care of organisms in the presence of a pathological condition, whether acute or chronic. All medications have the potential to cause side effects in patients, which can significantly impact their clinical state, either by exacerbating minor events or generating manifestations of greater severity. Therefore, healthcare professionals are tasked with identifying signs and symptoms related to clinical entities, including those caused by medication allergies and hypersensitivity, due to the increasing occurrence of adverse reactions to these drugs [1]. On the other hand, early and timely diagnosis of adverse drug reactions is of vital importance for comprehensive disease management and even for ensuring patient safety and establishing the most personalized treatment. For this reason, the study of medication allergy has been addressed nowadays, as it encompasses hypersensitivity, hyperreactivity, and immunologically mediated intolerance reactions through various mechanisms and clinical presentations. These reactions not only affect the patient's quality of life but also lead to treatment delays [2].

Hypersensitivity reactions to medications can be categorized based on timing (immediate or delayed), as well as the mechanisms and pattern of clinical manifestations. Similarly, they can be classified according to the Gel and Coombs system, which describes the predominant immunological mechanisms involved, identifying immediate-type reactions mediated by immunoglobulin E (IgE) antibodies, cytotoxic reactions mediated by immunoglobulin G (IgG) or immunoglobulin M (IgM)

N. Contreras-Puentes (✉) · M. Castro-Leones · B. Gutiérrez-Tovar · J. Mendoza-Galiz
GINUMED, School of Medicine, Cartagena D.T. y C., Corporación Universitaria Rafael Núñez, Bolívar, Colombia
e-mail: neyder.contreras@curnvirrtual.edu.co; m.castrol10@curnvirtual.edu.co; bgutierrezt10@curnvirtual.edu.co; jmendozag10@curnvirtual.edu.co

M. G. Múnera Gómez et al. (eds.), *Allergies, Poisoning and Intolerance to Common Substances*, https://doi.org/10.1007/978-3-031-93658-6_7

antibodies, immune complex reactions, and delayed-type hypersensitivity reactions mediated by cellular immune mechanisms, such as T-cell recruitment and activity [2, 3]. This is relevant due to the consolidation of potential mechanisms that notably explain the presence of underreported events and become significant in a particular therapeutic context.

In this chapter, we will explore the general foundations, mechanisms, and significance of the main allergic reactions, hypersensitivity, and toxicity associated with commonly used medications such as non-steroidal anti-inflammatory drugs (NSAIDs), beta-lactam antibiotics (BL), and neurological treatments like anticonvulsants.

Non-steroidal Anti-inflammatory Drugs (NSAIDs)

They are a broad and heterogeneous group of compounds that have been used for decades as highly effective analgesics. Their origins date back to 1828 with the isolation of salicin and the subsequent introduction of acetylsalicylic acid, known as aspirin, by Bayer in 1899 [4]. These are administered to treat a wide range of conditions, such as osteoarthritis, musculoskeletal diseases [5], due to their anti-inflammatory, analgesic, and antipyretic properties [6], furthermore, the over-the-counter availability of some formulations has allowed an increase in their usage over time. However, this easy accessibility has led to self-medication, resulting in the development of adverse drug reactions, including drug hypersensitivity, in 21–25% of cases [7].

In Colombia, by the year 2013, there were 1043 sanitary registrations corresponding to the group of NSAIDs in the Institute of Drug and Food Surveillance. Eight of the active ingredients in this pharmacological group have dual sales conditions (over the counter and prescription-only), accounting for 70% of the marketing authorizations [8].

Arachidonic Acid Metabolism and Related Pathways

Arachidonic acid (AA) is a polyunsaturated fatty acid [9], secreted by phospholipase A2 (PLA2) (resulting from the hydrolysis of the ester bond of phospholipids) or through phospholipase C (hydrolysis of phosphatidylinositol 4,5-bisphosphate) and phospholipase D (catalyzing phosphatidylcholine to generate phosphatidic acid or diacylglycerol (DAG), which is later hydrolyzed by DAG lipase to produce AA), releasing it from cell membrane phospholipids [10, 11]. And through the metabolism of different pathways, such as cyclooxygenase (COX) and lipoxygenase (LOX). The former allows the formation of thromboxane (TX) and prostaglandins (PG); the latter, leukotrienes (LT) and lipoxins (LX); and the third allows the synthesis of epoxyeicosatrienoic acids (EET) [12]. These products can be called eicosanoids, which are biologically active molecules produced by the oxidation of 20-carbon ω-3 or ω-6 fatty acids and are grouped into subcategories that include leukotrienes, lipoxins, hydroxyeicosatetraenoic acids, hydroxyeicosapentaenoic acids, eoxins, isoprostanes, resolvins, and prostanoids [13].

Cyclooxygenase (COX) Pathway

COX-1/2, also known as prostaglandin H synthase (PGHS), is a key enzyme involved in the metabolism of AA and the production of prostanoids, a term used for prostaglandin and thromboxane products. The constitutive enzyme COX-1 is expressed in all tissues and induces acute inflammation in response to brief exposure to lipopolysaccharide (LPS) stimulation, directing the cell to promote or suppress the biosynthesis of leukotrienes. COX-1 is also responsible for the expression of thromboxane A2 (TXA2), prostaglandin F2α, and prostaglandin D2. On the other hand, COX-2 is an inducible isoform found in macrophages in the kidneys and brain, which is involved in inflammatory processes and responsible to produce prostacyclin (PGI2) and prostaglandin E2 (PGE2). Once AA is released, it can be metabolized by two PGHS isoenzymes (PGHS-1 and PGHS-2). PGHS has two different but complementary enzymatic activities. One is the cyclooxygenase activity, which catalyzes the production of PGG2 from the introduction of two molecules of O_2 into AA. The other is the peroxidase activity, which promotes the reduction of PGG2 to PGH2 through a glutathione-dependent hydroperoxide reaction. COX initially metabolizes AA into the unstable PGG2 due to its cyclooxygenase function and then converts it to PGH2 through its peroxidase function. PGH2, like selective prostanoid synthases and isomerases in specific cells and tissues, is not stable and can easily generate many bioactive prostaglandins, such as prostaglandins D2, E2, F2α, I2, and TXA2, depending on the differential expression of synthases in tissues [14, 15] (see Fig. 7.1a).

For example, PGD2, PGE2, and PGI2 are potent vasodilators in the cardiovascular system, while TxA2 exhibits vasoconstriction in the same system. TxA2 plays an important role in platelet aggregation, while PGI2 shows anticoagulant properties. In the airway, TxA2 and PGF2α act as bronchoconstrictors; PGE2, PGI2, and PGF2α protect the gastric mucosa. Additionally, PGE2 and PGI2 have bronchodilator function and regulate blood flow and diuresis in compromised kidneys. Essentially, all the biological activities of these prostanoids depend on their binding to G protein-coupled cell surface receptors. The receptors for PGD2 are DP1 and DP2 receptors.

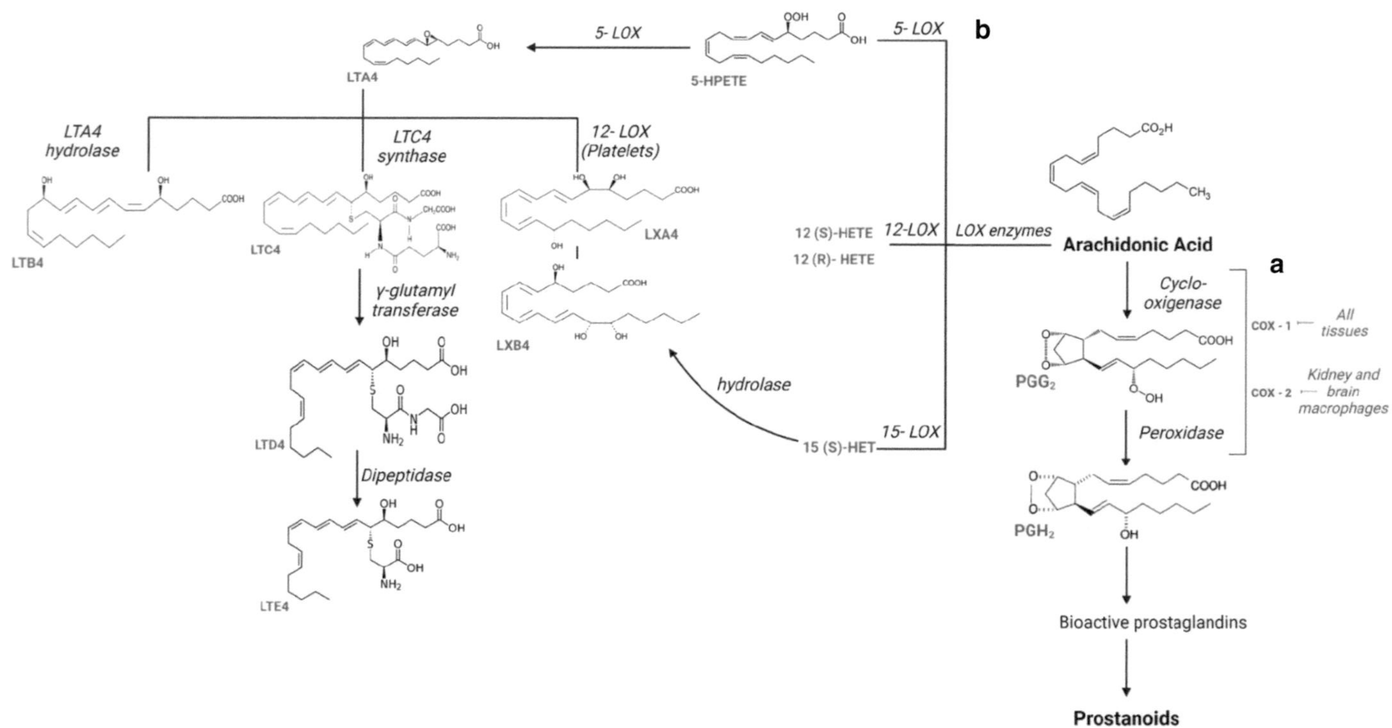

Fig. 7.1 The figure illustrates the metabolism of arachidonic acid through two main pathways: the COX pathway (**a**) and the LOX pathway (**b**). In the COX pathway, arachidonic acid is converted by cyclooxygenase into prostaglandins, which are bioactive lipids involved in inflammation and other processes. In the LOX pathway, lipoxygenase enzymes metabolize arachidonic acid into leukotrienes and lipoxins, which regulate immune responses and inflammation. Key intermediates include LTA4, which is further converted into leukotrienes (LTB4, LTC4, LTD4, LTE4), and lipoxins (LXA4, LXB4), with distinct biological effects. The pathways contribute to inflammation, immune regulation, and tissue homeostasis

Lipoxygenase (LOX) Pathway

The metabolites of the arachidonic acid 5-lipoxygenase (5-LOX) pathway regulate a series of functions in T cells, including proliferation, apoptosis, cytokine secretion, differentiation, chemotaxis, and a wide range of physiological processes, from inflammatory conditions such as asthma and allergies to diseases like cancer and viral infections [16]. The LOX enzymes insert oxygen at a molecular level into AA, forming 4 hydroperoxyeicosatetraenoic acids (HPETE; 5, 8, 12, and 15-HPETE) by the corresponding LOX enzymes (5, 8, 12, and 15-LOX). The HPETE are then reduced to monohydroxyeicosatetraenoic acids (HETE) by peroxidases or converted into biologically active compounds such as leukotrienes, lipoxins (LX), and hepoxilins [17].

AA forms 5-hydroperoxyeicosatetraenoic acid (5-HPETE) through dioxygenase, i.e., via homolytic cleavage and removal of hydrogen at the pro-S hydrogen on carbon-7 through the catalytic function of the enzyme 5-LOX. Thus, AA metabolites are converted to LTA4, due to the removal of the C10 hydrogen atom from 5-HPETE via the 5-LOX and dehydratase protein. LTA4 is unstable and is hydrolyzed by LTA4 hydrolase (LTA4H) to form the dihydroxy leukotriene LTB4. On the other hand, LTA4 is converted to LTC4 by the addition of glutathione via LTC4 synthase (LTC4S), which is then exported from the cell and converted to subsequent metabolites. The conversion of LTC4 by γ-glutamyl transferase results in the release of LTD4 and glutamic acid, where dipeptidase breaks the amide bond in LTD4 to synthesize LTE4 [11, 14].

On the other hand, 12-LOX and 15-LOX are involved in the generation of HETE and LX. The 12-LOX pathway is like the 5-LOX pathway. AA first favors 12-HPETE and 12-hydroxyeicosatetraenoic acid (12-HETE). However, 12-LOX can also convert 5(S)-HETE to 5(S),12(S)-dihydroxyeicosatetraenoic acid (-diHETE) and influence 15(S)-HETE to 14(R),15(S)-diHETE in leukocytes. These products ultimately lead to extraplatelet LTA4 formation. 5-LOX generates LTA4 in neutrophils, which is then transferred to the platelet, where 12-LOX subsequently generates LXA4 or LXB4. 15-LOX-1 and leukocyte 12-LOX can form 12(S)-HETE and 15(S)-HETE. When 15-LOX-2 metabolizes AA to produce only 15-HETE, 15-LOX-1 also metabolizes linoleic acid to synthesize hydroxyoctadecadienoic acid. Then, 15-HETE is rapidly converted to LXA4 or LXB4 by hydrolase [14, 17]. (See Fig. 7.1b).

Mechanism of Action

The main therapeutic actions of NSAIDs occur through the inhibition of the cyclooxygenase (COX) enzyme, of which there are 2 isoforms: COX-1 and COX-2 [18]. COX-1 produces prostaglandins and thromboxane A2 that control the mucosa in the gastrointestinal tract, renal homeostasis, platelet aggregation, and other physiological functions. COX-2 produces prostaglandins that are related to inflammation, pain, and fever [19]. In general terms, COX-1 is seen as the primary source of prostaglandins for general homeostatic regulation throughout the body, while COX-2 is more easily induced and is the dominant source of prostaglandins that mediate inflammation [20].

Some evidence supports the mechanism of NSAIDs, especially in studies of canine cerebral cortex cDNA library screening using a ≈ 1.0 kb fragment of previously cloned COX-1. These studies revealed two complete clones called COX-3 and partial COX-1a (PCOX-1a), both derived from the COX-1 gene. This has led to corroborating, in human tissue studies, the presence of high levels of COX-3 in the cerebral cortex and the heart. Furthermore, the ability to inhibit the activity of COX-1, COX-2, and COX-3 of common analgesic/antipyretic drugs and NSAIDs was evaluated, and it was found that COX-3 was significantly more sensitive to paracetamol, phenacetin, dipyrone, diclofenac, aspirin, and ibuprofen. This suggests that the COX-1 gene plays an integral role in pain and fever [21].

Hypersensitivity to NSAIDs

Hypersensitivity reactions can be induced or triggered by multiple NSAIDs that mainly inhibit COX-1 (multiple NSAID hypersensitivity or cross-reactivity) or by a single NSAID that causes a humoral or cellular immune response (single NSAID hypersensitivity or selective) [11]. In the case of the former, the reactions will be mediated by the release of inflammatory mediators following the inhibition of cyclooxygenase COX-1 [22], while the latter is responsible for reactions mediated by IgE or T cells [23].

Similarly, the European Academy of Allergy and Clinical Immunology (EAACI) distinguishes cross-reactive reactions (due to COX-1 inhibition) and selective hypersensitivity reactions (mediated by IgE or T cells) [24], providing a new classification that has been progressively adopted by many groups worldwide [25]: Cross-reactive reactions, Aspirin-Exacerbated Respiratory Disease (AERD), Aspirin-Exacerbated Cutaneous Disease (AECD), and Urticaria/Angioedema Induced by NSAIDs (UAI-NSAIDs) [26].

NSAIDs-Exacerbated Respiratory Disease (NERD)

Aspirin-exacerbated respiratory disease (NERD) is an important phenotype among the categories of cross-reactive hypersensitivity to NSAIDs [27]. This is defined as a chronic eosinophilic inflammatory disorder of the airways that occurs in patients with asthma and/or rhinosinusitis with nasal polyps, whose symptoms are exacerbated by NSAIDs [28]. It has been suggested that the prevalence of AERD in the general population is 0.3–0.9%. The prevalence is higher among patients with asthma (7%), chronic rhinosinusitis with nasal polyps (10%), or severe asthma (15%), and it reaches up to 30% among asthmatics with nasal polyposis [29]. According to Wongsa, C. et al., in a study conducted on patients with suggestive history of AERD with or without asthma, it was demonstrated that the most common agent was ibuprofen (60%), followed by mefenamic acid (40%), naproxen (20%), diclofenac (20%), and aspirin (20%). The most common NSAIDs may vary depending on the region because some are available over the counter in certain places, while in others, they are not [30].

After the ingestion of NSAIDs, symptoms appear within a period of 30–180 min, and their onset and severity are associated with the administered dose. Most patients develop symptoms with 60 mg of acetylsalicylic acid (ASA), but this range varies from 10 to 300 mg [31]. Clinically, AERD is characterized by a severe onset of nasal congestion followed by chronic rhinosinusitis and ultimately by the development of nasal polyps. Asthma is frequently, though not universally, associated with it. Additionally, nasal polyps (benign growths in the paranasal sinuses) can obstruct the airflow and cause difficulty in breathing and loss of sense of smell, making them a key feature for diagnosis. Similarly, the severity of sinus symptoms often correlates with the severity of asthma symptoms [32].

AERD is described with an eosinophilic and mast cell increase, along with the action of proinflammatory type 2 cytokines (T2). Furthermore, the active regulation of cysteinyl leukotrienes (cysLT) and other mediators such as prostaglandin D2 and PGE2 has been characterized [32, 33]. Therefore, the induction of LTC4, LTD4, and LTE4, together with binding to specific receptors CysLT1, CysLT2, and CysLT3, impacts the signaling of mechanisms such as bronchoconstriction, mucus production, vascular permeability, and accumulation of inflammatory cells [34]. In this way, LTC4 and LTD4 sensitize CysLT1R to induce smooth muscle contraction. Studies in humans and animal models have investigated the role of receptors such as CysLT2R in bronchoconstriction. Likewise, it has been addressed that LTE4, when interacting with CysLT1R and CysLT3R, stimulates mucin release and submucosal inflammation in the nasal mucosa in murine models [35].

Therefore, eosinophils, mast cells, basophils, and even macrophages are generally described as cellular responders to CysLT activation [34]. CysLT1R has been described to be expressed in mast cells, macrophages, and granulocytes, inducing a complex inflammatory reaction associated with the synthesis and signaling of LTC4, LTD4, and LTE4. Increases in CysLT enhance Th2 inflammation by directly activating Group 2 innate lymphoid cells (ILC2) through their interaction with CysLT1R and by upregulating the expression of other cytokine receptors such as thymic stromal lymphopoietin receptor (TSLPR), IL-33 receptor subunit, and suppression of tumorigenicity 2 (ST2) [35] (see Fig. 7.2).

Thus, in the studies conducted by Choi et al., it was observed that serum TGF-β1 levels were significantly higher in patients with AERD. Additionally, serum TGF-β1 levels and urinary LTE4 levels showed a positive correlation. In the presence of TGF-β1, the expression of LTC4S increased in peripheral eosinophils to produce LTE4, which subsequently induced eosinophil degranulation through the p38 signaling pathway. Similarly, studies in mice treated with TGF-β1 showed significantly

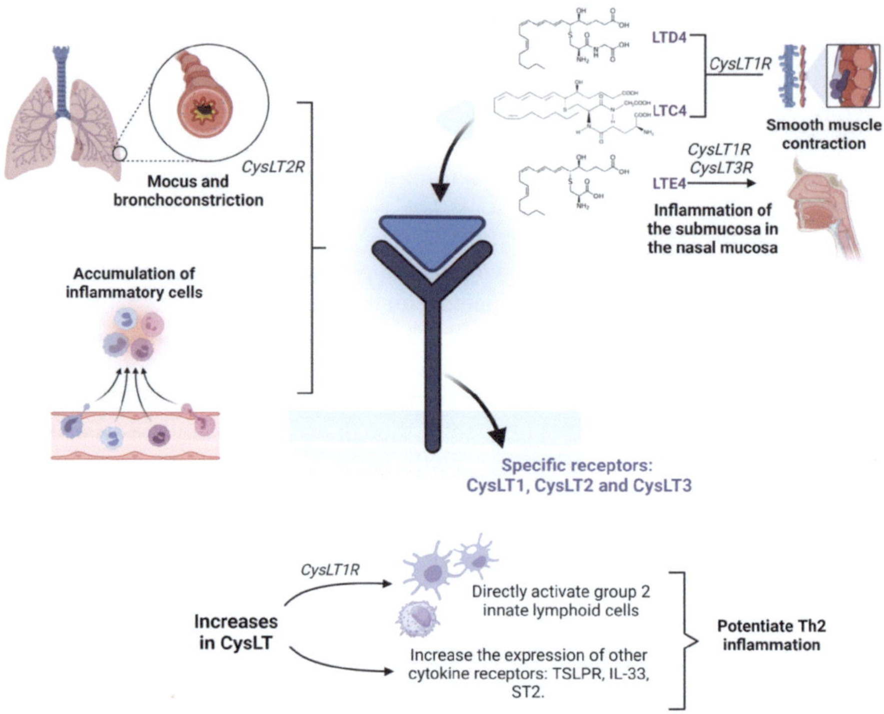

Fig. 7.2 Mechanisms of hypersensitivity associated with NSAID-exacerbated respiratory disease (AERD) and active CysLT

induced eosinophilia with higher production of LTE4 in lung tissues. Therefore, it is demonstrated that TGF-β1 in NERD patients may contribute to LTE4 production by enhancing LTC4S expression, which induces eosinophil degranulation, thus accelerating airway inflammation [36]. Klaewsongkram et al. indicated that in a Thai adult population with hypersensitivity to NSAIDs, elevated LTE4 levels following aspirin provocation suggested a diagnosis of cross-reactivity to NSAIDs, while baseline LTE4 levels did not distinguish between subjects tolerant and sensitive to NSAIDs. Moreover, persistently high uLTE4 levels despite clinical improvement in NSAID-sensitive patients after successful aspirin desensitization suggest that elevated leukotrienes alone cannot explain the pathogenesis of NSAID hypersensitivity reactions [37].

On the other hand, the presence of the clinical condition has been linked to an increase in PGD-2 (released from mast cells and eosinophils) which binds to prostanoid receptors to induce bronchoconstriction, and also binds to the homologous chemoattractant receptor expressed on TH2 cells (CRTH2) to induce chemotaxis and activate eosinophils, basophils, TH2 cells, and innate lymphoid cells (ILC2), accelerating type 2 airway inflammation [27]. Similarly, in studies conducted by Pal et al., it has been observed that PGE2, acting through its EP2 receptor, can inhibit the activation of eosinophils by aspirin. Salicylates will not activate eosinophils in individuals without AERD, as their persistent synthesis of PGE2 imposes restrictions on eosinophils (as well as on mast cells, basophils, and neutrophils adhering to platelets) [38].

It has been demonstrated that the binding of PGE2 to the EP2 receptor inhibits mast cell degranulation and prevents the migration of lung fibroblasts through increased intracellular cyclic AMP, ultimately acting as a brake for CysLT production. This contrasts with subjects with AERD, where reduced EP2 expression and function result in the paradoxical tendency for any PGE2 to only have proinflammatory EP1 and EP3 receptors, further driving an inflammatory cascade. Another restriction, along with the lower expression of EP2, is the higher affinity of PGE2 for the EP3 receptor. As a result, any available PGE2 will likely bind to the proinflammatory EP3 receptor [32, 38].

NSAIDs-Exacerbated Cutaneous Disease (NECD)

Also known as NSAIDs-Exacerbated Cutaneous Disease (NECD), this clinical condition accounts for 8% of cases of hypersensitivity reactions. Additionally, it has been linked to 10–30% of individuals identified with exacerbated chronic urticaria (ECU) associated with NSAIDs. Affected individuals are characterized by an exacerbation of the underlying disease with dermal involvement [39].

NSAIDs-Induced Urticaria/Angioedema (NIUA)

NSAIDs-induced urticaria/angioedema (NIUA) is a clinical phenotype characterized by hives and/or the development of angioedema in patients without chronic spontaneous urticaria (CSU) and represents the most common clinical entity [22].

For a long time, it has been recognized that the inhibition of COX-1 and the subsequent generation of inflammatory mediators in the arachidonic acid pathway play a central role in the etiopathogenesis of other hypersensitivity responses such as EREA and are also believed to be involved in ECEA. According to the study conducted by Doña et al., this hypothesis has been extended to UAIA, as they provided information on the levels of eicosanoids in urine, including LTE4 and 9α, 11β-PGF2 in UAIA patients [40]. On the other hand, thymic stromal lymphopoietin (TSLP), a cytokine produced by epithelial cells, has been implicated in initiating and maintaining the inflammatory response and has been shown to be overexpressed in the affected skin of patients with cutaneous diseases. According to the study conducted by Seron et al., only two SNPs in TSLP (rs1816678 and rs764917) showed a nominal association with NIUA, suggesting a potential role of TSLP in UAIA, although this needs to be confirmed [41].

The cutaneous reaction usually appears within 1 h after oral intake of the drug, but in some patients, it may develop within 1–6 h. In most cases, urticaria and angioedema appear simultaneously, AINE-induced angioedema) without urticaria or isolated periorbital angioedema has been observed. Typically, managing these patients involves avoiding the drug, and avoiding potentially reactive compounds (COX-1 inhibitors) would generally prevent the recurrence of urticaria/angioedema symptoms. However, if chronic intake of aspirin or other potent COX-1 inhibitors is necessary, desensitization to aspirin can be performed [42].

Toxicity Associated to Use of NSAIDs

The use of NSAIDs is associated with toxicity in various organs, such as the kidneys, liver, and gastrointestinal tract, affecting both the upper gastrointestinal tract (peptic ulcer disease) and the lower gastrointestinal tract (NSAID-induced enteropathy). The use of NSAIDs has been associated with an increased risk of clinical relapse in patients with inflammatory bowel disease (IBD) [43].

Quratulain et al., through a descriptive cross-sectional study, analyzed the preference, availability, and knowledge of the toxicity of NSAIDs and paracetamol, with a sample of 1000 respondents aged between 18 and 40 years. They found that the most used medication was mefenamic acid (n = 191, 40.8%), and paracetamol ranked second in the list of preferences (n = 146, 31.3%). Around 178 out of 467 (38.1%) used these medications for headache. Very few respondents knew about the toxic doses of the medications they used. Only 52 (11%) were aware that the increased bleeding tendency was the most common side effect of acetylsalicylic acid, and 129 (28%) knew about liver damage due to paracetamol toxicity [44].

It is known that NSAIDs cause damage at the gastric and duodenal levels, and they are also associated with drug-induced mortality and morbidity. In elderly patients, the use of these medications increases due to musculoskeletal disorders and cardiovascular diseases, resulting in complications such as peptic ulcers or upper gastrointestinal bleeding, attributed to the weakened gastric mucosa due to aging [45].

Nephrotoxicity can commonly occur and leads to acute kidney injury (AKI) in 1–5% of cases. Nephrotoxic effects mainly arise from two mechanisms: (1) acute tubulointerstitial nephritis (ATIN) due to an immune reaction, and (2) prerenal failure caused by reduced renal plasma flow [46]. Acute kidney injury (AKI) is nothing more than the abrupt reduction of renal function, which is characterized by oliguria of 0.5 ml/kg/h for >6 h, an increase in serum creatinine by ≥0.3 mg/dl or 1.5 times from baseline. Almost all NSAIDs can be associated with AKI; however, kidney damage caused by NSAID use is not common. Patients who suffer from AKI develop increased activity in two systems: the renin-angiotensin-aldosterone (RAA) system and the sympathetic nervous system. The increased activity of these systems contributes to vasoconstriction and, therefore, inhibits prostaglandin (PG) synthesis, in addition to the mechanism of COX blockade by NSAIDs. PGs are one of the factors that influence blood pressure due to their impact on vascular tone and the transport of fluids and electrolytes in renal structures. The alterations caused by

NSAIDs have minimal influence on blood pressure in normotensive patients; however, they could elevate blood pressure in hypertensive patients and attenuate the control with antihypertensive drugs [47].

Hepatotoxicity is another complication induced by NSAIDs, being less frequent than gastrointestinal damage, cardiovascular diseases, and renal insufficiency. Recent studies have found that drug-induced liver injury is a rare event. However, the severity lies in the widespread consumption and easy distribution of NSAIDs; in the United States alone, 30 million people take NSAIDs every year, thus opening up a potential threat of drug-induced liver damage. It is likely that the liver injury caused by most NSAIDs is idiosyncratic, and clinically evident liver injury is rare (approximately 1–10 cases per 100,000 prescriptions). Although sulindac and diclofenac are more commonly associated with hepatotoxicity, in particular, specific PGHS-2 NSAIDs are less likely to cause hepatotoxicity compared to nonselective NSAIDs. It is important to realize that NSAIDs can lead to two main clinical patterns of hepatotoxicity; the first being acute hepatitis (characterized by jaundice, nausea, and fever along with elevated serum levels of transaminases), while the other is chronic active hepatitis (characterized by serological and histopathological abnormalities) [48].

Diagnostic

It is common to observe hypersensitivity reactions to NSAIDs, but in some cases, reaching a correct classification and diagnosis can be tedious. Therefore, it is important to conduct a thorough medical history, including the time of symptom onset, a detailed description of the symptoms, and their correlation with each other. It is also essential to establish the number of previously reported episodes, evidence of cross-reactivity with other NSAIDs, the triggering dose of the ingested drugs, personal history of atopy, childhood polypectomy, or any characteristic underlying disease. Knowing the names of tolerated NSAIDs that patients are familiar with, the medications currently being consumed, and their current nasal status are also crucial aspects to consider. During the physical examination, it is essential to recognize specific patterns. For example, in skin involvement, it is important to specify if there is itching, redness, hives, or angioedema. Evaluating the involvement of mucous membranes and the extent of skin involvement is also vital in the diagnosis and classification of hypersensitivity reactions to NSAIDs [39, 49].

In addition, there are in vivo and in vitro tests that can guide the diagnosis, with the aspirin provocation test considered the gold standard for hypersensitivity reactions to NSAIDs [49]. This test consists of the administration through oral, intranasal, bronchial, or intravenous routes [50]. The aspirin provocation test consists of low-dose aspirin administration, and gradually increasing doses are given until a positive response is achieved. Usually, the doses start at 20–40 mg, and FEV1 is assessed every 30 min after the intake of each aspirin dose. Most symptoms occur between 45 and 100 mg within 30–60 min after the ingestion of the provoking dose [50, 51].

Other in vivo tests used include the skin prick test, which is only indicated if the medical history suggests NSAID-exacerbated respiratory disease (NERD); the intradermal test, but its sensitivity is not optimal, and there is a risk of subsequent systemic responses; and the patch test, which might be useful for non-immediate cutaneous drug hypersensitivity reactions (NIDHR). On the other hand, in vitro tests include assays for serum immunoglobulin E (IgE), total serum IgE, and specific IgE in serum complexes; although they may confirm the diagnosis, they have not been validated and are not recommended for clinical practice. Finally, basophil activation tests have limited diagnostic value and are not recommended either [52, 53].

On the other hand, the toxicity of NSAIDs can manifest at the gastrointestinal, hepatic, and renal levels. Typically, in the upper gastrointestinal tract, petechiae and ecchymosis may be found, but they may go undetected when asymptomatic or when patients present gastrointestinal symptoms without detectable lesions. In some cases, a complication can be the onset of NSAID-associated peptic ulcer disease. Meanwhile, in the lower gastrointestinal tract, there may be inflammation or increased intestinal permeability, iron-deficiency anemia, malabsorption, mucosal ulcers, among other conditions [54]. Similarly, there are diagnostic aids such as capsule endoscopy, enteroscopy, or endoscopy. However, these are not used routinely [55].

Similarly, it is important to evaluate liver function tests, as the elevation of transaminases can be crucial in cases of suspected hepatotoxicity due to NSAIDs [56]. On the other hand, NSAID-induced nephrotoxicity can lead to acute kidney injury, hydroelectrolytic imbalances (hyperkalemia and hyponatremia), and acute interstitial nephritis associated with nephrotic syndrome (clinically manifested by deteriorated renal function, hematuria, pyuria, and proteinuria) [57].

Treatment

After making a proper diagnosis, it is essential as the first measure for management to strictly avoid NSAIDs or seek alternatives. For example, if strong COX-1 inhibitors are avoided, weak COX-1 inhibitors, COX-2 inhibitors with some COX-1 effects, or COX-2 selective inhibitors can be provided. Additionally, associated symptoms should be treated, and complications should be prevented [25].

In the case of NSAID-exacerbated respiratory disease (NERD), the mainstay of treatment for both asthma and sinusitis includes inhaled steroids with or without a long-acting beta-agonist, intranasal steroids, and the use of systemic corticosteroids if necessary. On the other hand, in NSAID-exacerbated cutaneous disease (NECD) and urticaria and angioedema induced by NSAIDs (UAIA), the standard dose of second-generation H1 antihistamines is used, along with antihistamines with or without steroids, respectively [25, 49]. Similarly, desensitization to aspirin should be considered as an alternative in some subtypes of NSAID hypersensitivity, such as NSAID-exacerbated respiratory disease (NERD) and urticaria and angioedema induced by NSAIDs (UAIA), in patients for whom the medication is indispensable. This should be done considering the risk/benefit ratio, required dosage, and duration of treatment [25, 58].

Regarding the treatment of upper gastrointestinal tract lesions, two strategies are possible: 1. Combining NSAIDs with a gastroprotective treatment and 2. Using COXIBs (characterized by selective COX-2 inhibition). As for other pathologies, the treatment is less established; the only measure is to discontinue the use of NSAIDs. For example, in cases of hepatotoxicity, discontinuing the drug intake allows for resolution of the condition [54, 56].

β-lactam Antibiotics

Generalities of β-lactam Antibiotics

Beta-lactam antibiotics (BL) are one of the most widely used and highly significant classes of drugs globally due to their frequent use in both inpatient and outpatient settings. These are molecules naturally produced by various organisms belonging to the fungal kingdom, such as Penicillium spp. and Cephalosporium spp. Historically, the first member of this extensive group is penicillin G, which was discovered by Alexander Fleming in 1929. Later, in 1945, the Italian pharmacologist Giuseppe Brotzu identified the presence of other bactericidal compounds in crude filtrates of Cephalosporium. Based on this, the founder of the second group of β-lactams, Cephalosporin C, was created in 1964 by the laboratory of Howard Florey at Oxford [59, 60].

The classification of β-lactam antibiotics depends on their chemical nature in the fused ring at the pharmacological junction. Four classes make up the β-lactam family: penicillins, cephalosporins, carbapenems, and monobactams. The structural characteristics of all these classes are based on three key aspects: (1) the 2-azetidinone, which is a cyclic four-membered amide required for acylation; (2) the ring strain levels of the cyclic amide imposed by bicyclic structural designs; and (3) a critical acid residue for recognition by the active site of transpeptidase (see Fig. 7.3) [61, 62].

In 1974, Blumberg and Strominger, after reaching the conclusion that both penicillin and the D-Ala-D-Ala terminus of peptidoglycan (PGN) in gram-negative and gram-positive microorganisms were similar, proposed that all β-lactam antibiotics share the same mechanism of action, which inhibits the activity of penicillin-binding proteins (PBPs) and the formation of peptidic cross-links. It is believed that the inhibition of PBPs results in the formation of holes in the cell wall, which subsequently destabilizes the membrane and causes lysis in the microorganism [63, 64].

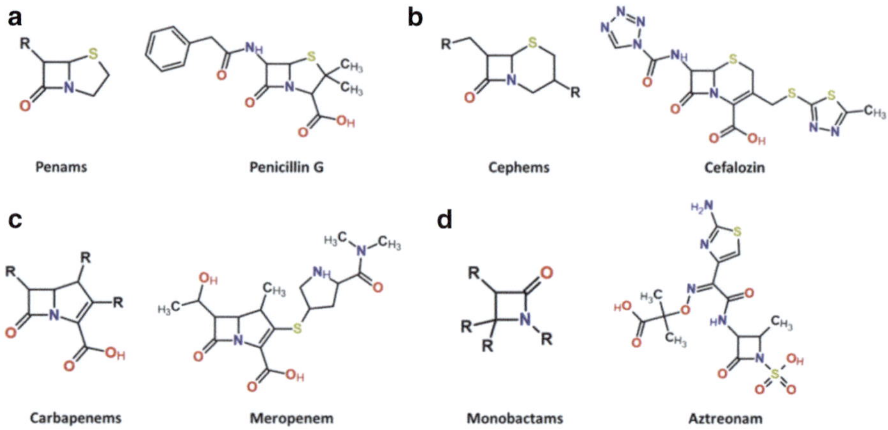

Fig. 7.3 Main β-lactam drugs used. In (**a**) penicillin, the β-lactam complex binds to a five-sulfur ring, forming the penam scaffold. (**b**) cephalosporin, the complex binds to a six-sulfur ring to generate the cephem scaffold. (**c**) in the carbapenem binds to a cyclopentene ring. (**d**) monobactams have no ring function to the β-lactam system

Hypersensitivity to β-lactam Antibiotics

Allergy to β-lactam antibiotics occurs in 7.92–14.5% of the hospital population, with penicillin and cephalosporins being the most common triggers. Hypersensitivity reactions induced by β-lactam antibiotics are mainly classified into immediate and non-immediate types, based on the time of onset after drug exposure. Immediate reactions involve an antibody-mediated pathway that increases the secretion of IgE, resulting in a rapid response within a few hours after exposure. On the other hand, non-immediate reactions are triggered through a T-cell-mediated response with an onset time ranging from 6 h to 4 weeks after medication. Clinical manifestations are diverse, including maculopapular exanthems and cutaneous adverse reactions (SCAR) ranging from 12.4% to 44.4%, as well as Stevens-Johnson syndrome (SJS), toxic epidermal necrolysis, and drug reaction with eosinophilia and systemic symptoms (DRESS) syndrome [65].

Hypersensitivity reactions are exaggerated or inappropriate responses to an antigen. Coombs and Gell classified these reactions into four types, which are immunologically mediated and have been associated with β-lactam antibiotics. Among them are Immediate hypersensitivity reactions are mediated by IgE (Type I), which manifests as urticaria, angioedema, wheezing, and hypotension. These are the most severe due to their rapid progression (within the first 72 h after contact with the medication). Type II reactions, which often cause hemolysis and thrombocytopenia. Type III reactions are mediated by immune complexes and typically cause glomerulonephritis and serum sickness. Type IV reactions are mediated by T-cells and often cause hepatitis, eosinophilia, contact dermatitis, and bullous rashes [66].

Penicillin Hypersensitivity

Penicillin allergy is the most frequent drug allergy in patients, affecting an estimated 10% of the global population. It is most associated with infection by methicillin-resistant *Staphylococcus aureus*, longer hospital stays, and increased patient mortality. Hypersensitivity tends to decrease over time, and 80% of patients become tolerant after a decade. Based on the clinical history, low-risk antecedents include isolated allergic symptoms, gastrointestinal symptoms, family history, itching without skin rashes, or remote unknown reactions. Moderate-risk history includes hives or other pruritic rashes and IgE-mediated reactions. High-risk history includes patients who have experienced anaphylaxis, positive penicillin skin test, and hypersensitivity to other beta-lactam antibiotics [67, 68].

Penicillin is characterized by its low molecular weight, which determines its immunogenic nature; however, the immune response is directed through complexes of degradation products or covalently formed adducts with self-proteins. The allergic components of penicillin are derived from the structure of the central beta-lactam ring or the side chains of the R-group. The beta-lactam ring spontaneously opens to form various breakdown products. The most frequent one is penicilloyl-polylysine or major allergenic determinant, which comprises 95% of the breakdown products. Among the remaining minor allergenic determinants are penicilloate and penilloate [69].

In type I reactions (mediated by IgE), dendritic cells bind to penicillin-bound proteins for the presentation to virgin CD4+ T cells. These T cells will differentiate into type 2 T cells, releasing interleukin 4 and 13, thereby inducing B cell differentiation and the production of specific IgE antibodies for penicillin. These IgE antibodies then bind to surface receptors on basophils and mast cells. Upon re-exposure, the response of these previously sensitized cells induces mast cell degranulation and the release of soluble inflammatory mediators such as tryptase, histamine, prostaglandins, and leukotrienes, leading to an immediate clinical manifestation with a high risk of anaphylaxis. In type II reactions, antibodies (IgM or IgG) target cell membrane structures of erythrocytes, leukocytes, or platelets, leading to the destruction or sequestration of cells, including hemolytic anemia and thrombocytopenia. On the other hand, type III reactions manifest with antibodies reacting to penicillin-binding proteins, generating soluble immune complexes, which trigger complement activity and deposition in small blood vessels, leading to neutrophil recruitment with the release of lytic proteins, causing tissue damage and local vascular inflammation, such as vasculitis, in small vessels and serum sickness. Finally, type IV reactions occur 6 h after penicillin administration or during treatment, after multiple exposures. An antigen-presenting cell processes drug-modified peptides and presents them at the HLA antigen binding site for recognition by T cell receptors (TCR) on CD4+ or CD8+ T cells, resulting in T cell activation, release of cytokines, and chemokines [70] (see Fig. 7.4).

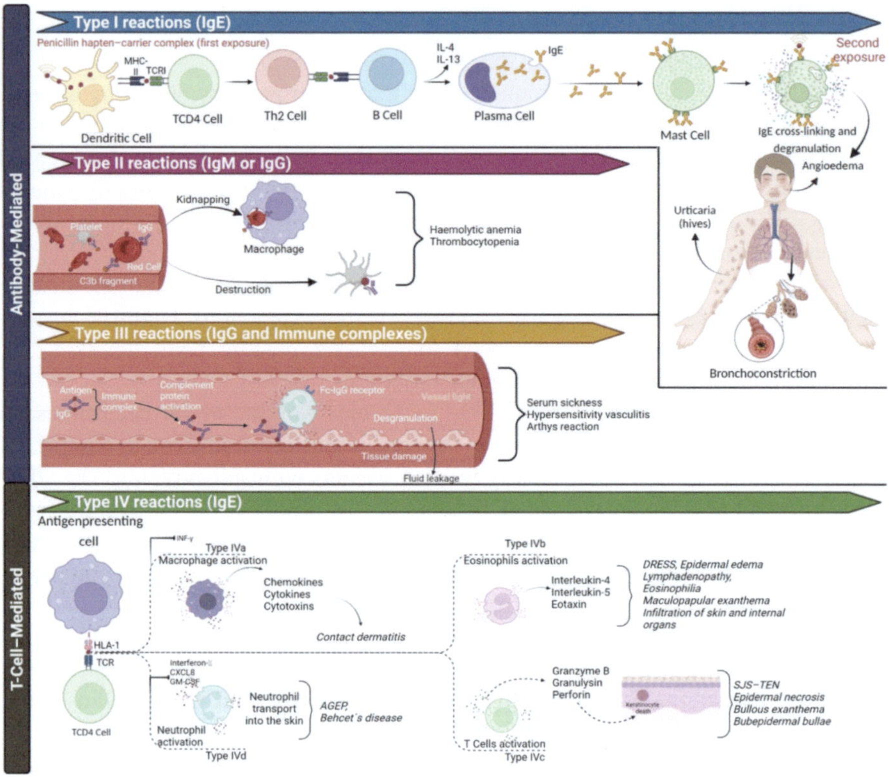

Fig. 7.4 Hyperreactivity associated with β-lactam drugs

Cephalosporin Hypersensitivity

It is estimated that the incidence of cephalosporin allergy is 1–3% of the general population. Cephalosporins are one of the leading causes of perioperative anaphylaxis and severe cutaneous adverse reactions. Allergic patients may tolerate cephalosporins with different R1 side chains but may react to other beta-lactam antibiotics with a common R1 side chain. Cephalosporins, like penicillins, are frequent causes of both immediate and delayed hypersensitivity reactions (HSR) phenotypes. Under physiological conditions, the beta-lactam ring is unstable and, in the case of penicillins, gives rise to major and minor determinants that covalently bind to host proteins, which have been well defined and used as testing strategies in clinical practice. Unlike penicillins, where the determinants are stable and identifiable, the determinants have not been reliably defined for cephalosporins, and the rate and efficiency with which cephalosporins form hapten-protein conjugates are comparatively lower than those of penicillins. Cephalosporins differ from penicillins both in their 6-membered dihydrothiazine ring and in the presence of an R2 group. Some evidence supports that the opening of the beta-lactam ring destroys the R2 side chain, leading to unstable conjugates and poorly identified fragmented determinants. Although IgE antibodies can theoretically bind to the beta-lactam ring, the carrier protein molecule, and the side chains, it is possible that the R1 side chain and the BL residue that covalently binds to host proteins are fundamental for immunogenicity [71, 72].

Toxicity Related to β-lactam Antibiotics

The selective toxicity of β-lactam antibiotics is attributed to their affinity for penicillin-binding proteins (PBPs) and the inhibition of bacterial cell wall biosynthesis, both of which are exclusive to prokaryotes. β-lactam antibiotics are generally considered safe; however, as the monitoring of plasma concentrations of β-lactam antibiotics becomes increasingly available, the risk of overexposure in patients is better identified. There is compelling evidence that toxicity can occur in intensive care unit (ICU) patients, even with β-lactam antibiotics [73]. In a retrospective analysis, patients treated with piperacillin, meropenem, or flucloxacillin have shown neurotoxicity effects during the use of any of these three antibiotics, as well as the development of nephrotoxicity during the use of piperacillin or meropenem at significantly higher mean minimum concentrations. This led to the concept of threshold minimum concentrations associated with a 50% risk of neurotoxicity or nephrotoxicity. On the other hand, septic patients in the ICU undergoing treatment with meropenem, ertapenem, piperacillin/tazobactam, ceftazidime, or cefepime have been evaluated, demonstrating that worsening neurological status was associated with increased minimum concentrations of piperacillin/tazobactam and meropenem [74, 75].

For this reason, reports of neurotoxicity have raised concerns about the development of myoclonus, encephalopathies, seizures, and nonconvulsive status epilepticus, possibly grounded in the structural similarity of β-lactam rings with the inhibitory neurotransmitter GABAA, both competitively and noncompetitively. Additionally, substitutions at positions 3 and 7 of the thiazolidine ring have been implicated in a potential epileptogenic mechanism [76]. On the other hand, other implicated mechanisms include decreased GABA release at neuronal terminals, reduced activity on benzodiazepine receptors, and an inductive effect of immune mediators and endotoxins that increase neurotoxicity [74].

On the contrary, evaluations in critically ill patients receiving conventional or higher-than-conventional doses of meropenem or piperacillin/tazobactam have indicated that there were no significant differences between the groups in the rates of various toxicities. Similarly, a single-center retrospective cohort study of 300 patients found that 5% of the patients experienced toxicity, but those patients did not have higher minimum concentrations than the patients who did not experience toxicity [77]. In general, β-lactam antibiotics are considered to have a high safety margin with relatively few adverse effects, even when used at high doses. Neurotoxicity is the most reported serious adverse effect of β-lactam antibiotics. Benzylpenicillin, cefepime, ceftazidime, and imipenem are considered high-risk β-lactams for neurotoxicity. It is known that renal insufficiency, excessive doses and/or concentrations, age, and a previous history of neurological disorders are predisposing factors [78].

Diagnosis

Beta-lactams are among the safest and most effective antibiotics; however, an increase in the prevalence of hypersensitivity has been found, limiting their use and resulting in the use of broad-spectrum antibiotics, which increases the risk of antimicrobial resistance [68]. The diagnosis of BL hypersensitivity is mainly based on patient risk staging (see Table 7.1) and diagnostic tests such as skin tests (ST), patch tests (PT) and drug reversal tests (DPT); however, their outcome depends on many factors such as the time interval between the reaction and the test, the severity of the reaction, and its chronology [79, 80].

Table 7.1 Patient risk staging [79]

Patient type	Type of reaction	Clinical manifestation
High-risk patients	Immediate reactions	Anaphylaxis Hypotension Laryngeal oedema Bronchospasm Urticaria and/or angioedema Generalized erythema
	Non-immediate reactions	Stevens-Johnson syndrome Toxic epidermal necrolysis Drug reaction (or exanthema) with eosinophilia and systemic symptoms Generalized bullous drug eruption Acute generalized exanthemata's pustulosis Linear IgA bullous dermatosis Severe maculopapular exanthema (MPE) Systemic vasculitis/serum sickness-like reaction Organ manifestations Drug-induced autoimmune diseases
Low-risk patients	Immediate reactions	Isolated generalized pruritus not requiring treatment Isolated gastrointestinal symptoms Local urticaria to parenteral administration
	Non-immediate reactions	Contact dermatitis Local infiltrative reaction to intramuscular administration Palmar exfoliative rash Fixed drug eruption Late onset urticaria Drug-related symmetrical intertriginous flexural exanthema

Table 7.2 Recommended nonirritant concentrations [79]

Haptene	Concentration
Benzyl Penicillyloyl-Poly-L-Lysine	$6{,}0 \times 10^{-5}$ Mol/L
Benzyl Penicilloyl-Octa-L-Lysine	$8{,}64 \times 10^{-5}$ Mol/L
Sodium benzylpenilloate	$1{,}5 \times 10^{-3}$ Mol/L
Benzylpenicillin	10,000 UI/mL
Amoxicillin and other semi-synthetic penicillin's	20 mg/mL
Cefepime	2 mg/ml
Other cephalosporins	20 mg/ml
Clavulanic acid	20 mg/ml
Aztreonam	2 mg/ml
Imipenem-cilastatin	0,5 mg/mL-0,5 mg/mL
Meropenem and ertapenem	1 mg/mL

Skin Tests (ST)

The skin tests are mediated by IgE, and there are two ways of performing them; (1) epicutaneous tests and (2) intradermal skin tests, if the epicutaneous test is negative. Nonirritant concentrations are used for these tests (see Table 7.2) [79, 80].

Patch Testing (PT)

It is a simple and safe diagnostic test; it should be used in patients experiencing severe skin reactions, such as Stevens-Johnson syndrome (SJS) and toxic epidermal necrolysis (TEN); in patients with suspected hypersensitivity to BL, it should be used as first line; in case it is positive, ST should be avoided; however, in case it is negative, interaction drug treatment (IDT) can be initiated, starting with a low concentration of the drug [79].

Drug Provocation Tests

A therapeutic dose of the drug will be administered under medical observation, and the current standard for identifying IgE-mediated allergies, the culprit BL will be administered in one, two, or three steps and monitored in each of these in 30–60 min [80]. DPT and TS have a predictive value of 99% when used to exclude IgE-mediated penicillin allergy [80].

Treatment

Despite the specific serum IgE evaluation for beta-lactams also showing reduced value in terms of both positive and negative predictability. The measurable detection of anti-beta-lactam IgE does not necessarily imply that exposure will result in an allergic response. Oral provocation testing is considered the gold standard for diagnosing beta-lactam allergy. In low-risk patients, a viable option would be to proceed directly with a gradual or single-step oral provocation. Gradual oral provocation involves administering 10% of the therapeutic dose. In the absence of symptoms, after 30–60 min, the remaining 90% of the therapeutic dose is given. This is followed by a minimum observation period of 60 min. In cases of intermediate risk, a penicillin skin test prior to challenge may be considered. Regarding patients with a history of allergy exclusively to penicillin, all beta-lactams can be administered as appropriate once successful amoxicillin provocation has been confirmed [81, 82].

The definitive resolution involves discontinuing the suspected antibiotic. In certain situations where the use of the antibiotic is essential due to a lack of more suitable alternatives, drug desensitization may be considered. Desensitization involves a reintroduction strategy of antibiotics in highly sensitized patients with the purpose of inducing tolerance. However, these individuals are still classified as allergic to the antibiotic. Rapid desensitization involves patients reaching the desired total dose of the medication through rapidly applied dose increments, usually within a 24-h period. On the other hand, gradual desensitization leads to patients reaching the desired total dose over a few days or weeks. Desensitization should be avoided if the initial reaction is potentially life-threatening, such as in the case of blistering rashes and SJS/NET, except for anaphylaxis [82, 83].

Anticonvulsants

Carbamazepine (CBZ)

Generalities, Metabolism, and Mechanism of Carbamazepine

It is an aromatic anticonvulsant drug related to tricyclic antidepressants, derived from the iminostilbene group, containing a carbamyl group at position 5, conferring potent anticonvulsant activity. It has a wide range of uses, from treating generalized tonic-clonic seizures, focal tonic-clonic seizures, and bilateral tonic-clonic seizures to trigeminal neuralgia and bipolar disorder treatment [84]. CBZ is characterized by the blockage of voltage-gated sodium channels (NaV), which are responsible for depolarizing the membrane during the propagation of action potentials across the surface of neuronal cells. These channels are expressed throughout the neuronal membrane, in dendrites, soma, axons, and nerve terminals [85], When NaV

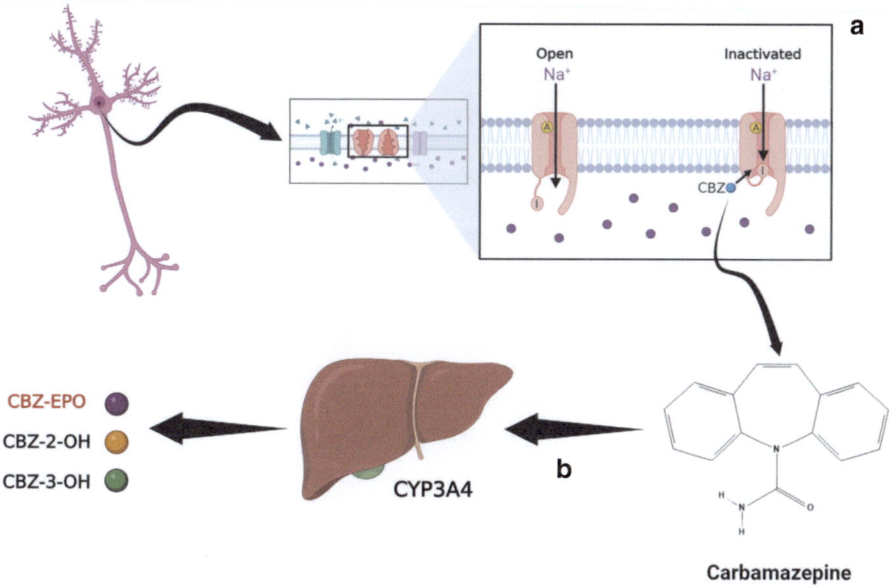

Fig. 7.5 Overview and mechanism of action of carbamazepine (CBZ). (**a**) Mechanism of action of CBZ. (**b**) Metabolic pathway and activation of CBZ metabolites

channels are at rest with the pore closed, membrane depolarization triggers their opening, allowing sodium entry for a few milliseconds, after which the channels become inactivated and the pore closes. This leads to both fast inactivation, occurring within milliseconds to terminate individual action potentials, and slow inactivation, which takes seconds to minutes and is likely to reduce membrane excitability [86] (Fig. 7.5a).

Metabolism mainly occurs in the liver by CYP3A4, converting it into carbamazepine 10,11-epoxide (CBZ-EPO), which is its active and potentially toxic metabolite. Additionally, there are other metabolites that contain a hydroxyl group, such as 2-hydroxycarbamazepine (CBZ-2-OH) and 3-hydroxycarbamazepine (CBZ-3-OH) [87] (see Fig. 7.5b). In acute doses, the initial elimination half-life is 25–65 h, decreasing to 4–17 h with repeated doses [88]. However, the use of this drug may lead to the presence of some side effects such as nausea, vomiting, dry mouth, hyponatremia, fatigue, tremors, and dizziness [89].

Allergy Associated with Carbamazepine

CBZ is associated with a high risk of adverse effects, mainly cutaneous effects, followed by organs such as the liver or bone marrow (see Table 7.3). However, the mechanisms of hypersensitivity reactions to carbamazepine are not well described. There are hypotheses that propose involvement of the immune system, which

Table 7.3 Main allergic or hypersensitivity reactions associated with the use of carbamazepine (CBZ)

Organ/system reaction	Reaction	
Skin	Maculopapular rash	
	Diffuse erythema	
	Exanthematous eruption	
	Urticaria	
	Purpuric Petechiae	
	Mucocutaneous syndrome	
	SJS/TEN	HLA-B*15:02
		HLA-B*15:21
	SJS	HLA-B*15:11
	DRESS	HLA-A*31:01
	Dermatomyositis	
	Eczema	
	Photosensitivity	
	Pustules	
	Psoriasiform and lichenoid reactions	
Bone marrow	Thrombocytopenia	
	Hypogammaglobulinemia	
	Leukopenia and neutropenia	
	Agranulocytosis	
	Aplastic anemia	
	Pure red cell aplasia	
	Acute lymphoblastic leukemia	
	Eosinophilia	

involves a complex interaction between drug metabolism, genetic variation of human leukocyte antigens (HLA), and immune system activation. This is due to reactive metabolites that can induce immune responses leading to pharmacological reactions. These reactive metabolites generate drug-modified peptides that are presented in the context of HLA molecules. Additionally, it requires a second cascade of co-stimulatory molecules on antigen-presenting cells (APC) thus, causing cellular damage leading to the release of damage-associated molecular patterns (DAMPs) [90]. On the other hand, the pathogenesis of hypersensitivity reactions raises hypotheses that describe genetic and host factors, especially the relationship between CBZ-specific CD4+ and CD8+ T cells and T cell receptors (TCR). This is possibly due to the proliferation of CD4+ and CD8+ T lymphocytes upon exposure to the drug through direct interaction of CBZ with HLA, leading to limited cytotoxicity. Additionally, this interaction stimulates the release of IFN-γ, IL-4, and IL-5 [91] (see Fig. 7.6).

At the cutaneous level, there is a wide range of clinical symptoms ranging from milder skin rashes to severe and potentially life-threatening syndromes. Scientific

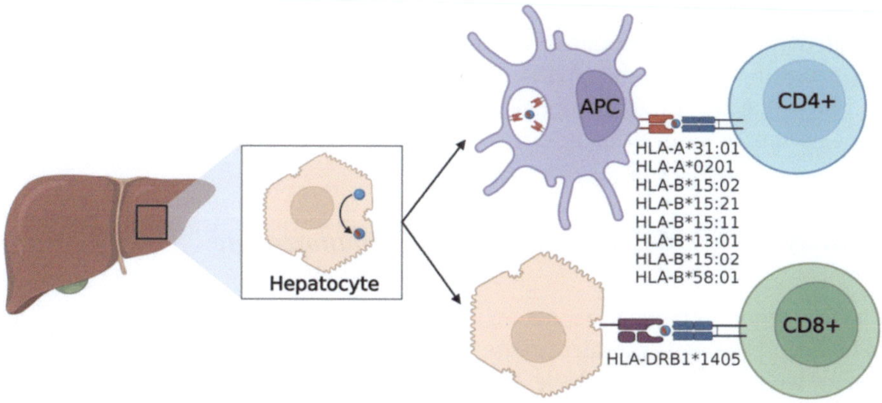

Fig. 7.6 Mechanisms of hypersensitivity and cross-reactivity associated with CBZ

evidence has established reports of severe cutaneous adverse reactions (SCAR), including drug reaction with eosinophilia and systemic symptoms (DRESS) syndrome, where skin rashes, changes in blood cell count, hepatitis, arthralgia, and lymphadenopathy are observed. Additionally, Stevens-Johnson syndrome (SJS), where skin detachment involves less than 10% of the body surface area, and toxic epidermal necrolysis (TEN) characterized by skin detachment in at least 30% of the body surface area [92, 93]. Many studies have demonstrated the association between HLA genotype and CBZ-induced SCAR; some HLA alleles have been reported as strong predictive markers. The most representative allele reported for CBZ-induced SJS/TEN is HLA-B*15:02, as well as HLA-B*15:21 [94]. There is also HLA-A*31:01, which has shown a significant association with DRESS and SJS [93]. The latter is also associated with HLA-B*15:11 [95]. Moreover, sporadic cases of secondary hemophagocytic lymphohistiocytosis have been described because of the activation of the DiHS/DRESS syndrome, which additionally exhibits a clinical pattern of patches or spots, blisters, and skin detachment, and seems to be linked to the HLA-B*1301 gene [96].

On the other hand, the use of CBZ has been associated with the development of maculopapular exanthema (EMP), characterized by macular or erythematous maculopapular lesions. Additionally, diffuse erythema, exanthematous rash, purpuric petechiae, and the development of a mucocutaneous syndrome have been reported [97]. The identification of this series of hypersensitivity responses, mainly associated with EMP, has been studied about the possible influence of HLA alleles in certain populations in China. It has been described that the frequencies of HLA-DRB1*1405 and HLA-A*0201 showed a higher expression in individuals with CBZ-EMP [98]. Similarly, in other populations such as Thai individuals, HLA-B*15:02 and HLA-B*58:01 alleles have been investigated, showing significant associations when compared with CBZ-tolerant groups, thus confirming their substantial involvement in the development of CBZ-induced EMP and DRESS [91].

Additionally, there are rare reactions such as dermatomyositis, eczema, photosensitivity, pustules, psoriasiform and lichenoid reactions, and anticonvulsant hypersensitivity syndrome (AHS). The latter consists of a triad of fever, skin rash, and involvement of internal organs, often affecting the liver, kidneys, central nervous system, or lungs [97].

Toxicity Associated with the Use of Carbamazepine

The first report of carbamazepine toxicity was first reported in 1967 and continues to be one of the most prevalent causes of anticonvulsant drug toxicity. It generally occurs with serum levels above 40 μg/mL in adult patients; however, it can be observed even with serum levels above 20 μ/mL. Severe toxicity has also been evidenced with ingestion of more than 50 mg/kg [84].

Acute carbamazepine intoxication can lead to stupor, hyperirritability, hallucinations, restlessness, and seizures at plasma concentration levels of 12–40 μg/mL. However, with progressively higher values above 40 μg/mL, the events intensify, leading to increased nausea, risk of status epilepticus, hematological toxicity in the form of thrombocytopenia, and even inducing thrombocytopenic purpura, leukopenia, neutropenia, and agranulocytosis, characterized by increased promyelocytes and myeloblasts and disappearance of neutrophils, aplastic anemia, acute lymphoblastic leukemia, or eosinophilia [99]. Among the mechanisms related to carbamazepine and its potential hematological toxicity, it is associated with the induction of oxidative stress through the generation of reactive oxygen species (ROS), which intervene in enzymatic regulation pathways and reduce regulatory components like glutathione. Additionally, metabolites involved in lipid peroxidation pathways in the erythrocyte membrane make it more vulnerable to hemolytic processes. On the other hand, the formation of CBZ metabolism compounds such as 10,11-epoxide has been described, which directly damages bone marrow progenitor cells, leading to aplastic anemia [100]. Also, hypersensitivity reactions such as dangerous skin reactions, eosinophilia, lymphadenopathy, and splenomegaly. A late complication is water retention, accompanied by a decrease in plasma osmolality and Na + concentration [101].

Lamotrigine (LTG)

Overview, Metabolism, and Mechanism of Lamotrigine

It is an anticonvulsant belonging to the group of aromatic antiepileptic drugs, derived from phenyltriazine [102]. It is used in the treatment of partial and generalized seizures, as well as for maintenance treatment in clinically stable patients with bipolar disorder. It has also been reported to have antidepressant effects in unipolar depression [103]. Lamotrigine is associated with low teratogenicity, which favors its use in women of childbearing age [104].

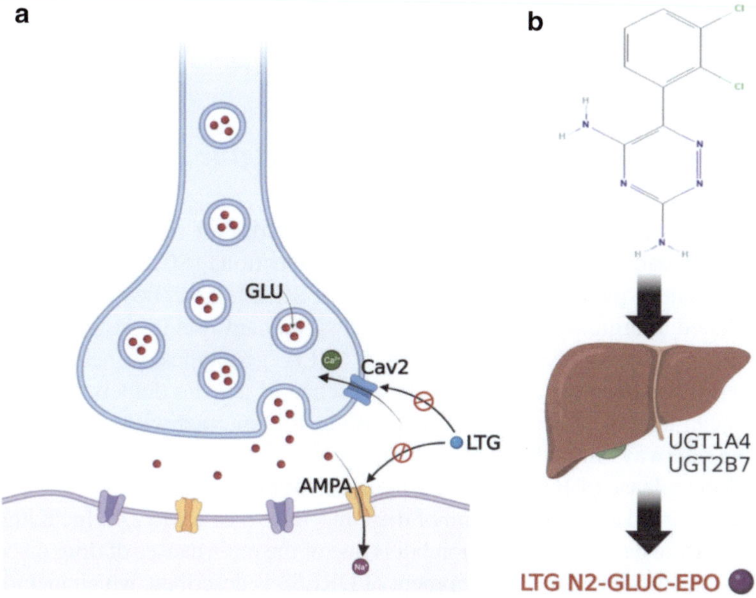

Fig. 7.7 Overview and mechanism of action of Lamotrigine (LTG). (**a**) Mechanism of action of LTG. (**b**) Metabolic pathway and activation of LTG metabolites

Like CBZ, lamotrigine is a blocker of NaV channels. However, it also inhibits the release of excitatory neurotransmitters. It mainly acts on cortical neurons because most of these neurons are excitatory and activate other neurons by releasing glutamate. Within the synaptic ionotropic glutamate receptors are the α-amino-3-hydroxy-5-methyl-4-isoxazolepropionic acid (AMPA) receptors, which belong to the main cationic channels responsible for rapid synaptic excitation. On the other hand, there are N-methyl-D-aspartate (NMDA) receptors, which are nonselective cationic channels activated by membrane depolarization coinciding with glutamate binding. Lamotrigine selectively blocks AMPA receptors [86, 104] (see Fig. 7.7a. In addition, LTG has immunomodulatory effects, which are relevant due to its allergic and hypersensitivity adverse effects. It has been reported that LTG can inhibit the secretion of IL-2, IL-1β, and TNF-α but not the secretion of IL-6, in human whole blood stimulated in vitro [105].

Lamotrigine is primarily metabolized in the liver, resulting in a half-life of a single dose of 24–30 h. The main metabolite of lamotrigine is lamotrigine N2-glucuronide (LTG N2-GLUC), which is formed by the UGT1A4 and UGT2B7 isoenzymes of uridine 5′-diphosphate-glucuronosyltransferase. Other metabolites, such as lamotrigine N2-oxide and lamotrigine N2-methyl, have also been characterized in low concentrations in humans [104]. Glucuronidation represents the main elimination pathway of LTG, with a half-life of elimination of about 24 h in monotherapy. The enzymatic activity of UDP-glucuronosyltransferase (UDPGT) will affect the levels of LTG and LTG N2-GLUC. The metabolite LTG N2-oxide appears to cause arene oxide toxicity, playing a significant role in the adverse effects of LTG, mainly rash and other cutaneous reactions [104, 106] (see Fig. 7.7b).

Allergy Associated with the Use of Lamotrigine

Lamotrigine is mainly associated with drug-related skin reactions, and in some cases, it can lead to severe cutaneous adverse reactions (SCAR). Therefore, it is crucial to identify patients with potential risk of SCAR. It has been described that T cell-mediated allergic reactions could play a significant role in the pathogenesis of these skin reactions; hence, the study of HLA genotypes is necessary [107]. Moreover, it has been described that the presence of genetic defects in detoxifying enzymes can lead to an increase in metabolites that interact with cellular proteins, activating pathways linked to T lymphocytes, which signal the generation of apoptosis and the release of IL-5, resulting in an eosinophilic increment [108].

There is a broad clinical spectrum of these reactions (see Table 7.4), including EMP, which is not a severe adverse reaction but is one of the main causes of drug discontinuation. On the other hand, the development of DRESS is described, which includes skin rash accompanied by fever, involvement of internal organs such as the liver, kidneys, lungs, nervous system, and eosinophilia [109]. Additionally, some evidence establishes cases of gastrointestinal disturbances associated with active colitis, where histopathological changes such as cryptitis, ulcerations, and eosinophilic infiltration of the lamina propria are observed [108]. Furthermore, rare and potentially life-threatening bullous reactions such as SJS (Stevens-Johnson syndrome) and TEN (toxic epidermal necrolysis) are also associated with lamotrigine. The HLA alleles HLA-DRB1*04:05 and HLA-DQB1*0401 are closely related to the occurrence of LTG-SCAR (Lamotrigine-Induced Severe Cutaneous Adverse Reactions) [107]. Another allele associated with the risk of LTG-SCAR is HLA-A*24:02 [110]. Similarly, the alleles HLA-A*02:07 and HLA-B*15:02 are also associated with the risk of LTG-SCAR in the Thai population. Additionally, the alleles HLA-A*33:03, HLA-B*15:02, HLA-A*31:01, and HLA-B*44:03 are related to the risk of developing LTG-EMP [102]. In the case of SJS, its pathogenesis is not fully understood, but widespread apoptosis of keratinocytes has been described. This event is believed to be caused by two hypotheses. The first hypothesis suggests that lamotrigine (LTG) and its metabolites can act as antigens for T cell receptors (TCR). The second hypothesis proposes that LTG and its metabolites noncovalently bind to the major histocompatibility complex, altering the binding groove and generating a self-peptide recognizable by T cells. This stimulates the release of Fas-Fas ligand, TNF-α, perforin-granzyme β, and granulysin, thereby mediating apoptosis. Additionally, other potential causes include the administration of valproic acid (VA), as it inhibits UDP-glucuronosyltransferases (UDPGT), leading to a diversion of LTG metabolism toward minor pathways such as CYP450, resulting in the production of toxic arene oxide metabolites. These metabolites form covalent bonds with DNA and RNA, causing cellular damage and acting as the initial trigger for the SJS reaction [111] (see Fig. 7.8).

Table 7.4 Major allergic or hypersensitivity reactions related to the use of Lamotrigine (LTG)

Organ/system	Reaction		
Skin	EMP		HLA-A*33:03 HLA-B*44:03
	RACS	SJS/TEN	HLA-B*15: 02
		EMP	HLA-A*24:02 HLA-A*31:01 HLA-DQB1*0401 HLA-A*02:07 HLA-B*15:02
		DRESS	
CNS	Decreased level of consciousness		
	Ataxia		
	Vertigo		
	Confusion		
	Agitation		
	Dysarthria		
	Nystagmus		
	Headache		
	Seizure		
	Ppsoclonus and myoclonus		
Cardiovascular	Arterial hypertension		
	Increased MAD in myocardial tissue		
	Brugada syndrome		
	QRS and QTc prolongation		
Respiratory	ARDS		
Lymphatic	Lymphadenopathy		

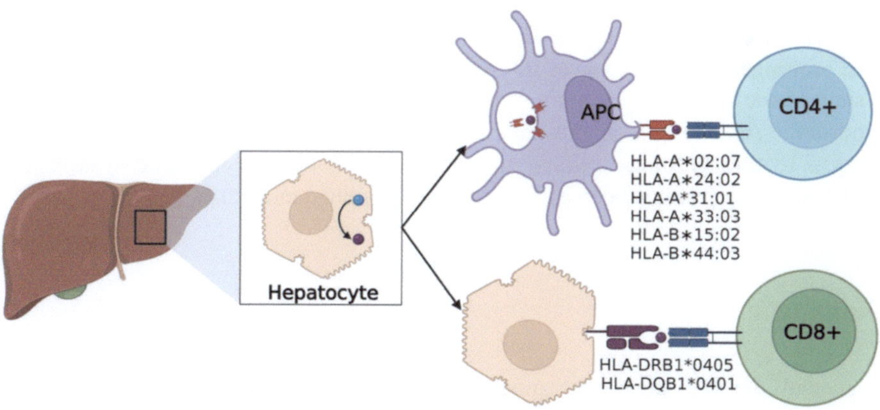

Fig. 7.8 Mechanisms of hypersensitivity and cross-reactivity associated with LTG

The hypersensitivity syndrome can also develop, which presents various clinical patterns such as skin rash, fever, lymphadenopathy, facial edema, eosinophilia, and abnormalities in liver function. In rare cases, it can even progress to multiorgan dysfunction [112].

Toxicity Associated with the Use of Lamotrigine

The main affected systems are the central nervous system (CNS) and the cardiovascular system, as the drug acts on channels responsible for initiating and propagating action potentials in nerves and muscles. At the CNS level, it can present with decreased level of consciousness and ataxia, followed by vertigo, confusion, restlessness, dysarthria, nystagmus, headache, seizures, and other findings associated with serotonin syndrome, given that LTG inhibits serotonin reuptake or is linked to LTG toxicity-induced encephalopathy [113]. Additionally, a significant pharmacological interaction with valproic acid (VA) has been identified. Therefore, in patients who are receiving lamotrigine as a baseline treatment, the administration of intravenous VA in emergency conditions, such as in cases of status epilepticus, can cause neurotoxicity. This is because VA reduces renal clearance, leading mainly to vertigo and nystagmus, and recently, the appearance of opsoclonus and myoclonus has been described [114, 115].

At the cardiovascular level, rare adverse effects such as disseminated intravascular coagulation (DIC) can occur due to LTG allergy based on immunoserological evidence [116]. High doses of LTG are associated with an increase in blood pressure and an elevation of malondialdehyde (MDA) in myocardial tissue [112]. Furthermore, it has been described that LTG has caused a phenocopy of Brugada syndrome (BS) type I in the ECG after the sodium channel block (SCB) test during BS evaluation [117]. There are also other changes in the ECG, such as QRS and QTc prolongation with R waves >3 mm in leads I and aVR [118]. Another affected system is the respiratory system, where LTG can cause acute respiratory distress syndrome (ARDS), which presents with pulmonary edema due to inflammatory damage to the alveolar-capillary membrane [119]. In the lymphatic system, the treatment with LTG has been associated with lymphadenopathies [120].

Diagnostic

In general, the pathogenesis of anticonvulsant hypersensitivity is the result of toxic metabolites that cause cell death or act as prohaptens to generate an immune response by binding to T lymphocyte receptors. In the case of skin rashes, CD4+ T cells are the main cell type involved [121]. On the contrary, SJS/TEN is a cytotoxic response mediated by specific CD8+ T cells, whereas DiHS/DRESS syndrome leads to massive activity of nonspecific T cells and immunoinflammatory responses [122].

Table 7.5 DiHS diagnostic criteria established by a Japanese consensus group and DRESS diagnostic criteria by RegiSCAR

(A) Diagnostic criteria for DIHS	(B) Diagnostic criteria for DRESSS
1. Maculopapular rash developing >3 weeks after starting a limited number of drugs.	1. Acute rash
2. Prolonged clinical symptoms after discontinuation of the offending drug	2. Reaction suspected to be related to a drug
3. Fever (>38C)	3. Hospitalization
4. Hepatic abnormalities (ALT>100 U/L)	4. Fever (>38C)
5. Leukocyte abnormalities (at least one present)	5. Laboratory abnormalities (at least 1 present)
A. Leukocytosis (>11,109 /L)	A. Lymphocytosis or lymphopenia
B. Atypical lymphocytosis (>5%)	B. Thrombocytopenia

The diagnosis is confirmed by the presence of the above seven criteria (typical DIHS) or all five (1–5) (atypical DIHS)
It can be replaced by involvement of other organs, such as kidney involvement

The diagnosis of these conditions is challenging but usually made through the anamnesis, physical examination, and sometimes skin biopsy. In the case of DiHS/DRESS syndrome, for DiHS specifically, it can be based on the diagnostic criteria established by the Japanese Research Committee on Severe Cutaneous Adverse Reactions (J-SCAR) (Table 7.5A) [123] and the RegiSCAR group for DRESS (Table 7.5B) [124].

Treatment

The first 3 criteria are necessary for the diagnosis, along with the presence of 3 out of the remaining 4. Regarding management, early recognition of the clinical picture and discontinuation of the suspected drug are the most important therapeutic measures. Whenever possible, it is essential to inquire with the patient and/or their relatives about details of all medications taken, including their chronology and dosage [125]. Systemic corticosteroids have been accepted as the treatment of choice to improve the clinical symptoms of DiHS/DRESS in the acute phase, such as dexamethasone (15–20 mg per day) or prednisolone (0.5–0.7 mg/kg/day), for periods of up to 8 weeks. However, it is important to note that these medications should be gradually tapered over 3–6 months to avoid relapses after clinical stabilization and normalization of laboratory results or therapy with antihistamines. Additionally, it may be possible to replace the offending drug with a safer alternative, such as valproate or clonazepam [124, 126]. For the case of SJS/TEN, supportive care in a burn intensive care unit is always the first-line treatment. This care is aimed at preventing fluid loss, preventing infections, and promoting skin healing using a variety of different biological dressings, lidocaine anesthetic gel, chlorhexidine mouthwash, or dexamethasone eye drops [121]. In some cases of TEN, the use of methylprednisolone pulses is recommended, with daily doses of 1 g for 3 days. In severe cases, intravenous human immunoglobulin has also been recommended at a dose of 2 g/kg/day for 5 days [126].

Conclusions

Medications are crucial elements in the well-being of the population, playing a role in prevention, diagnosis, and treatment. However, continuous administration can induce a series of secondary and adverse events that significantly impact individual health. Most of these responses are associated with immune system dysregulation, leading to clinically manifested allergic reactions, hypersensitivity, and toxicity. Thus, commonly used drugs like nonsteroidal anti-inflammatory drugs, beta-lactam antibiotics, and anticonvulsants can induce various degrees of reactions affecting different organs. In this chapter, we have described the general and molecular basis of the main manifestations associated with the use of these drugs, such as exacerbated cutaneous diseases, eosinophilic and systemic alterations, maculopapular exanthema, Stevens-Johnson syndrome, and central disorders like ataxia, vertigo, and seizures, among others. Additionally, a significant approach was made to the main events associated with toxicity due to the use of these agents, mainly highlighting cardiovascular, renal, hematological, and neurotoxic alterations.

Glossary

Glossary of Acronyms

AA Arachidonic acid
AAS Acetylsalicylic acid (Aspirin)
NSAID Nonsteroidal Anti-inflammatory Drugs
AMPA α-Amino-3-hydroxy-5-methyl-4-isoxazolepropionic acid
BL β-Lactams
CBZ Carbamazepine
CBZ-EPO Carbamazepine 10,11-epoxide
CBZ-2-OH 2-Hydroxycarbamazepine
CBZ-3-OH 3-Hydroxycarbamazepine
CLI2 Group 2 Innate Lymphoid Cells
COX Cyclooxygenase
CPA Antigen-Presenting Cells
CysLT Cysteinyl Leukotriene
CysLT1R Cysteinyl Leukotriene Receptor 1
CysLT2R Cysteinyl Leukotriene Receptor 2

CysLT3R Cysteinyl Leukotriene Receptor 3
DAMPs Damage-Associated Molecular Patterns
DAG Diacylglycerol
diHETE Dihydroxyeicosatetraenoic acid
DRESS Drug Reaction with Eosinophilia and Systemic Symptoms
NECD NSAID-Exacerbated Cutaneous Disease
EET Epoxyeicosatrienoic acids
EMP Maculopapular Exanthema
EREA NSAID-Exacerbated Respiratory Disease
ERO Reactive Oxygen Species
GABA Gamma-Aminobutyric Acid
HETE Hydroxyeicosatetraenoic acids
HLA Human Leukocyte Antigens
HPETE Hydroperoxyeicosatetraenoic acids
IL-33 Interleukin 33
LOX Lipoxygenase
LPS Lipopolysaccharides
LT Leukotriene
LTA4 Leukotriene A4
LTC4 Leukotriene C4
LTD4 Leukotriene D4
LTE4 Leukotriene E4
LTG Lamotrigine
LX Lipoxins
LXA4 Lipoxin A4
LXB4 Lipoxin B4
NaV Voltage-Activated Sodium Channels
NERD NSAID-Exacerbated Respiratory Disease
NET Toxic Epidermal Necrolysis
PBP Penicillin-Binding Proteins
PGN Peptidoglycan
PLA2 Phospholipase A2
PG Prostaglandins
PGE2 Prostaglandin E2
PGHS Prostaglandin H synthase
PGI2 Prostacyclin
SCAR Severe Cutaneous Adverse Reactions
SJS Stevens-Johnson Syndrome
ST2 Suppressor of Tumorigenicity 2
TCR T Cell Receptors
TGF-β1 Transforming Growth Factor Beta 1
TSLPR Thymic Stromal Lymphopoietin Receptor
TX Thromboxanes
TXA2 Thromboxane A2
UAIA Urticaria/Angioedema Induced by NSAIDs

UCE Chronic Urticaria Exacerbated
UCI Intensive Care Unit
UDPGT UDP-glucuronosyltransferase
12-LOX 12-Lipoxygenase
15-LOX 15-Lipoxygenase
5-LOX 5-Lipoxygenase

Glossary of Terms

β-lactam Partially bactericidal antibiotics that have a central β-lactam ring core, inhibit bacterial wall synthesis by interfering with peptidoglycan synthesis through transpeptidation blockade.

Arachidonic acid Unsaturated essential ω-6 fatty acid and a precursor in the biosynthesis of prostaglandins, thromboxanes, and leukotrienes. It is found in the liver, brain, glandular organs, and animal fat deposits, in small amounts in human fat deposits, and is a drawback.

Nonsteroidal anti-inflammatory drug (NSAID) A chemically heterogeneous group of various drugs, primarily anti-inflammatory, analgesic, and antipyretic, which act by competitively and stereospecifically inhibiting the enzyme cyclooxygenase.

Carbamazepine An antiepileptic and analgesic that reduces glutamate release, stabilizes neuronal membranes, and depresses dopamine and norepinephrine turnover.

Cephalosporins Cephalosporins are bactericidal antibiotics with a beta-lactam ring attached to a dihydrothiazoline ring that interferes with the synthesis of the peptidoglycan component of the bacterial cell wall, through binding to penicillin-binding protein (PBP) and inactivation of endogenous autolysin inhibitors.

Cyclooxygenase An enzyme that catalyzes the synthesis of prostaglandins through the oxidation of arachidonic acid.

NSAID-Exacerbated Cutaneous Disease (NECD) Hypersensitivity reactions produced by ASA or any other NSAID that manifest as urticaria and/or angioedema in patients with chronic spontaneous urticaria.

NSAID-Exacerbated Respiratory Disease (NERD) A reaction characterized by bronchial obstruction symptoms, dyspnea, and nasal congestion/rhinorrhea in patients with pre-existing airway disease (asthma/rhinosinusitis/nasal polyps) after the ingestion of aspirin and other NSAIDs that inhibit cyclooxygenase-1 (COX-1).

Maculopapular rash Papules on an erythematous base.

Lamotrigine A triazine-derived antiepileptic that blocks voltage-dependent sodium channels, blocking hyperexcitable neurons and inhibiting pathological glutamate and aspartate release.

Lipoxygenase A family of enzymes containing a non-heme iron group responsible for catalyzing the addition of molecular oxygen to polyunsaturated fatty acids. It is involved in the metabolic pathway of synthesizing leukotrienes from arachidonic acid.

Leukotriene Fatty acids derived from the oxidative metabolism of arachidonic acid through the 5-lipoxygenase pathway.

Monobactams Antibiotics with a monocyclic beta-lactam ring that inhibit bacterial wall synthesis.

Toxic Epidermal Necrolysis (TEN) A severe adverse skin reaction characterized by widespread necrosis of keratinocytes in the context of inappropriate immune activation by certain drugs or their metabolites, with skin detachment involving at least 30% of the body surface.

Penicillin Drug with common chemical core (6-aminopenicillanic acid) containing an essential beta-lactam ring for their biological activity. Peptidoglycan synthesis is inhibited due to transpeptidation blockage.

Peptidoglycan Chains of amino sugars linked together by short peptide chains to form a mesh surrounding the plasma membrane, providing shape and osmotic resistance to bacteria.

Penicillin-Binding Proteins (PBPs) β-lactam-binding proteins found in the cytoplasmic membrane of bacteria. There are six well-known types, and four of them, 1a, 1b, 2, and 3, are responsible for the antimicrobial mechanism of action of β-lactams.

Prostaglandins A group of substances belonging to the 20-carbon fatty acids (eicosanoids), containing a cyclopentane ring, and constituting a family of cellular mediators with diverse and often opposing effects.

Severe Cutaneous Adverse Reactions (SCAR) Delayed hypersensitivity reactions that include Stevens-Johnson Syndrome (SJS), Toxic Epidermal Necrolysis (TEN), Drug Reaction with Eosinophilia and Systemic Symptoms (DRESS), due to extensive rash and the possibility of systemic symptoms.

Stevens-Johnson Syndrome A severe adverse skin reaction where skin detachment involves no more than 10% of the body surface.

Drug Reaction with Eosinophilia and Systemic Symptoms (DRESS) A hypersensitivity reaction characterized by skin rash, hematologic abnormalities, lymphadenopathy, and involvement of organs such as the liver, kidney, and lungs.

Thromboxane A metabolite of arachidonic acid, thromboxane A2 is the primary in vivo thromboxane synthesized by platelets when activated by other aggregating compounds. It causes arteriolar constriction and is a potent inducer of platelet aggregation.

Th2 Lymphocyte Secretes IL-4, IL-5, and IL-10, promoting humoral immunity and inducing antibody production.

References

1. Broyles AD, Banerji A, Barmettler S, et al. Practical guidance for the evaluation and management of drug hypersensitivity: specific drugs. J Allergy Clin Immunol Pract. 2020;8:S16–S116.
2. Warrington R, Silviu-Dan F, Wong T. Drug allergy. Allergy Asthma Clin Immunol. 2018;14:60.
3. Dykewicz MS, Lam JK. Drug hypersensitivity reactions. Med Clin North Am. 2020;104:109–28.
4. Baldo BA, Pham NH. Non-steroidal anti-inflammatory drugs. In: Drug allergy; 2021. p. 439–71.
5. Bettiol A, Marconi E, Vannacci A, et al. Effectiveness of ibuprofen plus paracetamol combination on persistence of acute musculoskeletal disorders in primary care patients. Int J Clin Pharm. 2021;43:1045–54.
6. Ricciotti E, Laudanski K, FitzGerald GA. Nonsteroidal anti-inflammatory drugs and glucocorticoids in COVID-19. Adv Biol Regul. 2021;81:100818.
7. Jurado-Escobar R, Doña I, Bogas-Herrera G, et al. Platelet-adherent leukocytes associated with cutaneous cross-reactive hypersensitivity to nonsteroidal anti-inflammatory drugs. Front Pharmacol. 2020;11:594427.
8. Vista de Determinación del riesgo de daño hepático relacionado a los medicamentos AINEs en pacientes con Chikun-Gunya y Zika. https://revistas.unicartagena.edu.co/index.php/cbiomedicas/article/view/3041/2573. Accessed 5 Sept 2022.
9. Hoxha M. What about COVID-19 and arachidonic acid pathway? Eur J Clin Pharmacol. 2020;76(11):1501–4.
10. Das UN. Arachidonic acid and other unsaturated fatty acids and some of their metabolites function as endogenous antimicrobial molecules: a review. J Adv Res. 2018;11:57–66.
11. Trinh HKT, Pham LD, Le KM, et al. Pharmacogenomics of hypersensitivity to nonsteroidal anti-inflammatory drugs. Front Genet. 2021;12 https://doi.org/10.3389/FGENE.2021.647257/FULL.
12. Pedrosa S, Cabezas MÁ. Ácidos Grasos Omega 3 en el tratamiento del dolor Prostaglandins PGE 2 PGD 2 PGF 2αa.
13. Jane Mitchell CA, Kirkby NS, Mitchell JA. Eicosanoids, prostacyclin and cyclooxygenase in the cardiovascular system, vol. 176; 2018. p. 1038. https://doi.org/10.1111/bph.v176.8/issuetoc.
14. Wang T, Fu X, Chen Q, et al. Arachidonic acid metabolism and kidney inflammation. Int J Mol Sci. 2019;20 https://doi.org/10.3390/IJMS20153683.
15. Hanna VS, Hafez EAA. Synopsis of arachidonic acid metabolism: a review. J Adv Res. 2018;11:23–32.
16. Baek SJ, Eling T. Novel applications of NSAIDs: insight and future perspectives in cardiovascular, neurodegenerative, diabetes and cancer disease therapy. Int J Mol Sci. 2021;22:6637.
17. Wang B, Wu L, Chen J, et al. Metabolism pathways of arachidonic acids: mechanisms and potential therapeutic targets. Signal Transduct Target Ther. 2021;6:1–30.
18. Thong BY-H. Nonsteroidal anti-inflammatory drug hypersensitivity in the Asia-Pacific. Asia Pac Allergy. 2018;8 https://doi.org/10.5415/APALLERGY.2018.8.E38.
19. Wongrakpanich S, Wongrakpanich A, Melhado K, et al. A comprehensive review of nonsteroidal anti-inflammatory drug use in the elderly. Aging Dis. 2018;9:143.
20. Li X, Mazaleuskaya LL, Ballantyne LL, et al. Genomic and lipidomic analyses differentiate the compensatory roles of two COX isoforms during systemic inflammation in mice. J Lipid Res. 2018;59:102.
21. Chandrasekharan NV, Dai H, Roos KLT, et al. From the cover: COX-3, a cyclooxygenase-1 variant inhibited by acetaminophen and other analgesic/antipyretic drugs: cloning, structure, and expression. Proc Natl Acad Sci USA. 2002;99:13926.

22. Jurado-Escobar R, Doña I, Triano-Cornejo J, et al. Genetic variants in cytosolic phospholipase A2 associated with nonsteroidal anti-inflammatory drug–induced acute Urticaria/Angioedema. Front Pharmacol. 2021;12:667824.
23. Pérez-Sánchez N, Doña I, Bogas G, et al. Evaluation of subjects experiencing allergic reactions to non-steroidal anti-inflammatory drugs: clinical characteristics and drugs involved. Front Pharmacol. 2020;11:503.
24. Doña I, Pérez-Sánchez N, Eguiluz-Gracia I, et al. Progress in understanding hypersensitivity reactions to nonsteroidal anti-inflammatory drugs. Allergy. 2020;75:561–75.
25. Blanca-Lopez N, Soriano V, Garcia-Martin E, et al. NSAID-induced reactions: classification, prevalence, impact, and management strategies. J Asthma Allergy. 2019;12:217.
26. Hermans MAW, Otten R, Karim AF, et al. Nonsteroidal anti-inflammatory drug hypersensitivity: not always an allergy! Neth J Med. 2018;76(2):52–9.
27. Woo SD, Luu QQ, Park HS. NSAID-exacerbated respiratory disease (NERD): from pathogenesis to improved care. Front Pharmacol. 2020;11 https://doi.org/10.3389/FPHAR.2020.01147.
28. Andersén H, Ilmarinen P, Honkamäki J, et al. NSAID-exacerbated respiratory disease: a population study. ERJ Open Res. 2022;8:00462. https://doi.org/10.1183/23120541.00462-2021.
29. Suikkila A, Hafrén L, Lyly A, et al. Patient-reported control of asthma, nasal polyposis, and middle-ear symptoms in NSAID-exacerbated respiratory disease. Front Allergy. 2021;2:716169.
30. Wongsa C, Sompornrattanaphan M, Tantilipikorn P, et al. Allergy and Immunology Clinical characteristics and aspirin desensitization in Thai patients with a suggestive history of NSAID-exacerbated respiratory disease. Asian Pac J Allergy Immunol. 2022; https://doi.org/10.12932/ap-150619.
31. Eraso I, Sangiovanni S, Morales EI, et al. Aspirin desensitization in NSAID-exacerbated respiratory disease and its outcomes in the clinical course of asthma: a systematic review of the literature and meta-analysis. PLoS One. 2021;16:e0247871. https://doi.org/10.1371/JOURNAL.PONE.0247871.
32. Sehanobish E, Asad M, Barbi M, et al. Aspirin actions in treatment of NSAID-exacerbated respiratory disease. Front Immunol. 2021;12:2460.
33. Rhyou HI, Nam YH, Park HS. Emerging biomarkers beyond leukotrienes for the Management of Nonsteroidal Anti-inflammatory Drug (NSAID)-exacerbated respiratory disease. Allergy Asthma Immunol Res. 2022;14:153.
34. Miyata J, Fukunaga K, Kawashima Y, et al. Dysregulated metabolism of polyunsaturated fatty acids in eosinophilic allergic diseases. Prostaglandins Other Lipid Mediat. 2020;150:106477.
35. Rusznak M, Peebles RS. Prostaglandin E2 in NSAID-exacerbated respiratory disease: protection against cysteinyl leukotrienes and group 2 innate lymphoid cells. Curr Opin Allergy Clin Immunol. 2019;19:38.
36. Choi Y, Sim S, Lee DH, et al. Effect of TGF-β1 on eosinophils to induce cysteinyl leukotriene E4 production in aspirin-exacerbated respiratory disease. PLoS One. 2021;16:e0256237. https://doi.org/10.1371/JOURNAL.PONE.0256237.
37. Klaewsongkram J, Buranapraditkun S, Mongkolpathumrat P, et al. Clinical characteristics, urinary leukotriene E4 levels, and aspirin desensitization results in patients with NSAID-induced blended reactions. Allergy Asthma Immunol Res. 2021;13:229.
38. Pal K, Ramsden M, Shim YM, et al. Suppression of aspirin-mediated eosinophil activation by prostaglandin E2: relevance to aspirin/NSAID hypersensitivity. Ann Allergy Asthma Immunol. 2019;123:503.
39. Wöhrl S. NSAID hypersensitivity—recommendations for diagnostic work up and patient management. Allergo J Int. 2018;27:114.
40. Doña I, Jurado-Escobar R, Perkins JR, et al. Eicosanoid mediator profiles in different phenotypes of nonsteroidal anti-inflammatory drug-induced Urticaria. Allergy. 2019;74:1135–44.
41. Plaza-Seron MDC, Blanca-Lopez N, Perez-Sanchez N, et al. Genetic variants of thymic stromal lymphopoietin in nonsteroidal anti-inflammatory drug-induced Urticaria/angioedema. Int Arch Allergy Immunol. 2016;169:249–55.

42. Kowalski ML, Woessner K, Sanak M. Approaches to the diagnosis and management of patients with a history of nonsteroidal anti-inflammatory drug-related urticaria and angioedema. J Allergy Clin Immunol. 2015;136:245–51.
43. Hijos-Mallada G, Sostres C, Gomollón F. NSAIDs, gastrointestinal toxicity and inflammatory bowel disease. Gastroenterología y Hepatología (English Edition). 2022;45:215–22.
44. Zamir Q, Nadeem A. Non-steroidal anti-inflammatory drugs vs. paracetamol: drug availability, patients' preference and knowledge of toxicity. J Ayub Med Coll Abbottabad. 2016;28:746–9.
45. Chu SJ, Yoon KT, Kim JS. Prevention of non-steroidal anti-inflammatory drug-induced peptic ulcers. Korean J Gastroenterol/Taehan Sohwagi Hakhoe chi. 2020;76:232–7.
46. Clavé S, Rousset-Rouvière C, Daniel L, et al. The invisible threat of non-steroidal anti-inflammatory drugs for kidneys. Front Pediatr. 2019;7:520.
47. Drożdżal S, Lechowicz K, Szostak B, et al. Kidney damage from nonsteroidal anti-inflammatory drugs—myth or truth? Review of selected literature. Pharmacol Res Perspect. 2021;9 https://doi.org/10.1002/prp2.817.
48. Bindu S, Mazumder S, Bandyopadhyay U. Non-steroidal anti-inflammatory drugs (NSAIDs) and organ damage: a current perspective. Biochem Pharmacol. 2020;180:114147.
49. Yeung WYW, Park HS. Update on the management of nonsteroidal anti-inflammatory drug hypersensitivity. Yonsei Med J. 2020;61:4.
50. Enrique Carrasco-Ortega C, Enrique Morales-Ríos J, Huerta-López JG. La enfermedad respiratoria exacerbada por aspirina y la desregulación de los mastocitos. Aspirin-exacerbated respiratory disease and mast cell dysregulation. 2021;30:19–23.
51. Dominas C, Gadkaree S, Maxfield AZ, et al. Aspirin-exacerbated respiratory disease: a review. Laryngoscope Investig Otolaryngol. 2020;5:360–7.
52. Menon B, Patel V. Indian guidelines for diagnosis of respiratory allergy. Indian J Allergy Asthma Immunol. 2023; https://doi.org/10.4103/0972-6691.367373.
53. Kowalski ML, Makowska JS. Seven steps to the diagnosis of NSAIDs hypersensitivity: how to apply a new classification in real practice? Allergy Asthma Immunol Res. 2015;7:312–20.
54. Hijos-Mallada G, Sostres C, Gomollón F. AINE, toxicidad gastrointestinal y enfermedad inflamatoria intestinal. Gastroenterol Hepatol. 2022;45:215–22.
55. Bielsa-Fernández MV, Tamayo-de la Cuesta JL, Lizárraga-López J, et al. Consenso mexicano sobre diagnóstico, prevención y tratamiento de la gastropatía y enteropatía por antiinflamatorios no esteroideos. Rev Gastroenterol Mex. 2020;85:190–206.
56. González-Olivares C, Martínez AA. Protocolo de evaluación de la afectación hepática en las enfermedades inmunológicas. Medicine – Programa de Formación Médica Continuada Acreditado. 2020;13:277–81.
57. Martín NS, Miguel PM. Afectación renal por fármacos, medios diagnósticos y tóxicos. Medicine – Programa de Formación Médica Continuada Acreditado. 2019;12:4840–8.
58. Luis J, Saldaña C. Desensibilización con AAS: Utilidad e indicaciones.
59. Tooke CL, Hinchliffe P, Bragginton EC, et al. β-Lactamases and β-Lactamase inhibitors in the 21st century. J Mol Biol. 2019;431:3472–500.
60. de Rosa M, Verdino A, Soriente A, et al. The odd couple(S): an overview of beta-lactam antibiotics bearing more than one pharmacophoric group. Int J Mol Sci. 2021;22:1–21.
61. Hamon A, Bastides F, Lefort A. Betalactámicos. EMC – Tratado de Medicina. 2021;25:1–7.
62. Turner J, Muraoka A, Bedenbaugh M, et al. The chemical relationship among Beta-lactam antibiotics and potential impacts on reactivity and decomposition. Front Microbiol. 2022;13:642.
63. Lima LM, da Silva BNM, Barbosa G, et al. β-lactam antibiotics: an overview from a medicinal chemistry perspective. Eur J Med Chem. 2020;208:112829.
64. Wong F, Wilson S, Helbig R, et al. Understanding beta-lactam-induced lysis at the single-cell level. Front Microbiol. 2021;12:2085.
65. Lumkul L, Chuamanochan M, Nochaiwong S, et al. Genetic association of beta-lactams-induced hypersensitivity reactions: a protocol for systematic review and meta-analysis. Genes (Basel). 2022;13 https://doi.org/10.3390/genes13040681.

66. Vardakas KZ, Kalimeris GD, Triarides NA, et al. An update on adverse drug reactions related to β-lactam antibiotics. Expert Opin Drug Saf. 2018;17:499–508.
67. Chua KYL, Vogrin S, Bury S, et al. The penicillin allergy Delabeling program: a multicenter whole-of-hospital health services intervention and comparative effectiveness study. Clin Infect Dis. 2021;73:487–96.
68. Shenoy ES, Macy E, Rowe T, et al. Evaluation and management of penicillin allergy: a review. JAMA. 2019;321:188–99.
69. Har D, Solensky R. Penicillin and Beta-lactam hypersensitivity. Immunol Allergy Clin N Am. 2017;37:643–62.
70. Felix MMR, Aun MV, de Menezes UP, et al. Allergy to penicillin and betalactam antibiotics. Einstein. 2021;19:eMD5703.
71. Chaudhry SB, Veve MP, Wagner JL. Cephalosporins: a focus on side chains and β-lactam cross-reactivity. Pharmacy. 2019;7:103.
72. Khan DA, Banerji A, Bernstein JA, et al. Cephalosporin allergy: current understanding and future challenges. J Allergy Clin Immunol Pract. 2019;7:2105–14.
73. Dalhoff A. Selective toxicity of antibacterial agents—still a valid concept or do we miss chances and ignore risks? Infection. 2021;49:29–56.
74. Roger C, Louart B. Beta-lactams toxicity in the intensive care unit: an underestimated collateral damage? Microorganisms. 2021;9:1505.
75. Hurkacz M, Dobrek L, Wiela-Hojeńska A. Antibiotics and the nervous system—which face of antibiotic therapy is real, Dr. Jekyll (neurotoxicity) or Mr. Hyde (neuroprotection)? Molecules. 2021;26 https://doi.org/10.3390/molecules26247456.
76. Chow KM, Hui AC, Szeto CC. Neurotoxicity induced by beta-lactam antibiotics: from bench to bedside. Eur J Clin Microbiol Infect Dis. 2005;24:649–53.
77. Cusumano JA, Klinker KP, Huttner A, et al. Towards precision medicine: therapeutic drug monitoring-guided dosing of vancomycin and β-lactam antibiotics to maximize effectiveness and minimize toxicity. Am J Health Syst Pharm. 2020;77:1104–12.
78. Veiga RP, Paiva JA. Pharmacokinetics–pharmacodynamics issues relevant for the clinical use of beta-lactam antibiotics in critically ill patients. Crit Care. 2018;22:1–34.
79. Romano A, Atanaskovic-Markovic M, Barbaud A, et al. Towards a more precise diagnosis of hypersensitivity to beta-lactams – an EAACI position paper. Allergy. 2020;75:1300–15.
80. Blumenthal KG, Peter JG, Trubiano JA, et al. Antibiotic allergy. Lancet. 2019;393:183.
81. Jeimy S, Ben-Shoshan M, Abrams EM, et al. Practical guide for evaluation and management of beta-lactam allergy: position statement from the Canadian Society of Allergy and Clinical Immunology. Allergy Asthma Clin Immunol. 2020;16:95. https://doi.org/10.1186/s13223-020-00494-2.
82. Thong BYH. Update on the management of antibiotic allergy. Allergy Asthma Immunol Res. 2010;2:77–86.
83. Iuliano S, Senn L, Moi L, et al. Management of beta-lactam antibiotics allergy: a real-life study. Front Allergy. 2022;3 https://doi.org/10.3389/falgy.2022.853587.
84. Nasif MA, Falana HH, Hamed HKH, et al. Severe carbamazepine toxicity treated with continuous Venovenous hemofiltration at Palestine medical complex: two case reports. Int Med Case Rep J. 2022;15:205–8.
85. Sills GJ, Rogawski MA. Mechanisms of action of currently used antiseizure drugs. Neuropharmacology. 2020;168:107966.
86. Kobayashi K, Endoh F, Ohmori I, et al. Action of antiepileptic drugs on neurons. Brain Dev. 2020;42:2–5.
87. Nowak PM, Mitoraj M, Sagan F, et al. Differentiation of isomeric metabolites of carbamazepine based on acid-base properties; experimental vs theoretical approach. J Chromatogr A. 2021;1651:462275. https://doi.org/10.1016/j.chroma.2021.462275.
88. Eryavuz Onmaz D, Abusoglu S, Ozturk B, et al. Determination of serum carbamazepine and its metabolite by validated tandem mass spectrometric method and the effect of carbamazepine on various hematological and biochemical parameters. J Pharm Biomed Anal. 2021;205:114299.

89. Fricke-Galindo I, Llerena A, Jung-Cook H, et al. Carbamazepine adverse drug reactions. Expert Rev Clin Pharmacol. 2018;11:705–18.
90. Kato R, Ijiri Y, Hayashi T, et al. The 2-Hydroxyiminostilbene metabolite of carbamazepine or the supernatant from incubation of hepatocytes with carbamazepine activates inflammasomes: implications for carbamazepine-induced hypersensitivity reactions. Drug Metab Dispos. 2019;47:1093–6.
91. Sukasem C, Chaichan C, Nakkrut T, et al. Association between HLA-B alleles and carbamazepine-induced maculopapular exanthema and severe cutaneous reactions in Thai patients. J Immunol Res. 2018;2018:2780272.
92. Simper GS, Gräser LS, Celik AA, et al. The mechanistic differences in HLA-associated carbamazepine hypersensitivity. Pharmaceutics. 2019;11 https://doi.org/10.3390/pharmaceutics11100536.
93. Genin E, Chen DP, Hung SI, et al. HLA-A*31:01 and different types of carbamazepine-induced severe cutaneous adverse reactions: an international study and meta-analysis. Pharmacogenomics J. 2014;14:281–8.
94. Jaruthamsophon K, Tipmanee V, Sangiemchoey A, et al. HLA-B∗15:21 and carbamazepine-induced Stevens-Johnson syndrome: pooled-data and in silico analysis. Sci Rep. 2017;7:45553.
95. Wang Q, Sun S, Xie M, et al. Association between the HLA-B alleles and carbamazepine-induced SJS/TEN: a meta-analysis. Epilepsy Res. 2017;135:19–28.
96. Guo Z, Gao J, Fan X, et al. Carbamazepine-induced DiHS/DRESS syndrome leading to hemophagocytic lymphohistiocytosis in a woman carrying the HLA-B*1301 gene. Pharmazie. 2021;76:23–6.
97. Mehta M, Shah J, Khakhkhar T, et al. Anticonvulsant hypersensitivity syndrome associated with carbamazepine administration: case series. J Pharmacol Pharmacother. 2014;5:60–3.
98. Li L-J, Hu F-Y, Wu X-T, et al. Predictive markers for carbamazepine and lamotrigine-induced maculopapular exanthema in Han Chinese. Epilepsy Res. 2013;106:296–300.
99. Lorigados Pedre L, Sarria Kessel MA, Pavón Fuentes N, et al. Toxicidad Hepática Y Hematológica De La Carbamazepina En La Epilepsia Farmacorresistente Y Su Relación Con Variables Clínicas. Panorama Cuba y Salud. 2021;16:41–9.
100. Padda J, Khalid K, Syam M, et al. Association of anemia with epilepsy and antiepileptic drugs. Cureus. 2021;13:1–5.
101. Himmerkus N, Sievers B, Bleich M. Carbamazepine affects water and electrolyte homoeostasis in rat-similarities and differences to vasopressin antagonism. Nephrol Dial Transplant. 2012;27:3790–8.
102. Koomdee N, Pratoomwun J, Jantararoungtong T, et al. Association of HLA-A and HLA-B alleles with lamotrigine-induced cutaneous adverse drug reactions in the Thai population. Front Pharmacol. 2017;8 https://doi.org/10.3389/fphar.2017.00879.
103. Ostadhadi S, Ahangari M, Nikoui V, et al. Pharmacological evidence for the involvement of the NMDA receptor and nitric oxide pathway in the antidepressant-like effect of lamotrigine in the mouse forced swimming test. Biomed Pharmacother. 2016;82:713–21.
104. Yang H, Zhang D, Mei S, et al. Simultaneous determination of plasma lamotrigine, lamotrigine N2-glucuronide and lamotrigine N2-oxide by UHPLC-MS/MS in epileptic patients. J Pharm Biomed Anal. 2022;220:115017.
105. Abu-Rish EY, Elhayek SY, Mohamed YS, et al. Evaluation of immunomodulatory effects of lamotrigine in BALB/c mice. Acta Pharma. 2017;67:543–55.
106. Vázquez M, Maldonado C, Guevara N, et al. Lamotrigine-valproic acid interaction leading to Stevens–Johnson syndrome. Case Rep Med. 2018;2018:5371854.
107. Ito A, Shimada H, Ishikawa K, et al. Association between HLA-DRB1∗0405, -DQB1∗0401 and -DQA1∗0303 alleles and lamotrigine-induced cutaneous adverse drug reactions. A pilot case-control study from Japan. J Affect Disord. 2015;179:47–50.
108. Parsi M, Daniel C. Lamotrigine-induced DRESS syndrome manifesting as 'eosinophilic colitis': an uncommon presentation of a very uncommon condition. Cureus. 2020;12:e7570.

109. Han SH, Hur MS, Youn HJ, et al. Drug reaction with eosinophilia and systemic symptom syndrome induced by lamotrigine. Ann Dermatol. 2017;29:206–9.
110. Li W, Wang J, Lin H, et al. HLA-A*24:02 associated with lamotrigine-induced cutaneous adverse drug reactions: A systematic review and meta-analysis. Medicine (United States). 2020;99:e23929. https://doi.org/10.1097/MD.0000000000023929.
111. Edinoff AN, Nguyen LH, Fitz-Gerald MJ, et al. Lamotrigine and Stevens-Johnson syndrome prevention. Psychopharmacol Bull. 2021;51:96–114.
112. Yıldız A, Vardı N, Parlakpınar H, et al. Effects of low- and high-dose Valproic acid and lamotrigine on the heart in female rats. Cardiovasc Toxicol. 2022;22:326–40.
113. Lambea Gil Á, Caldú Agud R, Rodríguez Gascón D, et al. Encephalopathy secondary to lamotrigine toxicity. Neurologia (Barcelona, Spain). 2020;35:439–40.
114. Zouari R, Bouchaala W, ben Nsir S, et al. Opsoclonus myoclonus induced by lamotrigine toxicity. Seizure. 2021;91:247–50.
115. Jung I, Shin JH, Kim J. Gaze-evoked nystagmus associated with valproic acid-induced lamotrigine toxicity. Clin Neurol Neurosurg. 2020;196:106013.
116. Takeshima M, Ishikawa H, Shimizu T, et al. Lamotrigine-induced disseminated intravascular coagulation with anticonvulsant hypersensitivity syndrome: a case report. Psychosomatics. 2016;57:540–2.
117. Leong KMW, Seligman H, Varnava AM. Proarrhythmogenic effects of lamotrigine during ajmaline testing for Brugada syndrome. HeartRhythm Case Rep. 2017;3:167–71.
118. Chavez P, Casso Dominguez A, Herzog E. Evolving electrocardiographic changes in lamotrigine overdose: a case report and literature review. Cardiovasc Toxicol. 2015;15:394–8.
119. Takeshima M, Ishikawa H, Shimizu T. Acute respiratory distress syndrome and lamotrigine: a case report. Psychosomatics. 2017;58:313–6.
120. Pomeroy SJ, Ndikumana R, Cavanagh JP. Lamotrigine induced lymphadenopathy: case report and literature review. Int J Pediatr Otorhinolaryngol. 2017;98:82–4.
121. Mani R, Monteleone C, Schalock PC, et al. Rashes and other hypersensitivity reactions associated with antiepileptic drugs: a review of current literature. Seizure. 2019;71:270–8.
122. Błaszczyk B, Lasoń W, Czuczwar SJ. Antiepileptic drugs and adverse skin reactions: an update. Pharmacol Rep. 2015;67:426–34.
123. Mizukawa Y, Hirahara K, Kano Y, et al. Drug-induced hypersensitivity syndrome/drug reaction with eosinophilia and systemic symptoms severity score: a useful tool for assessing disease severity and predicting fatal cytomegalovirus disease. J Am Acad Dermatol. 2019;80:670–678.e2.
124. Shiohara T, Mizukawa Y. Drug-induced hypersensitivity syndrome (DiHS)/drug reaction with eosinophilia and systemic symptoms (DRESS): an update in 2019. Allergol Int. 2019;68:301–8.
125. Bonilla-Bustos AB, Moribe-Quintero IC, Gómez-Urrego JF. Síndrome de DRESS inducido por carbamazepina: una grave reacción de hipersensibilidad retardada. Alergia, Asma e Inmunología Pediátricas. 2022;31:51–7.
126. Marín JA, Ortega MA, Sánchez IP, et al. Síndrome de hipersensibilidad a medicamentos con exantema, eosinofilia y síntomas sistémicos inducido por carbamazepina. Biomedica. 2017;37:150–7.

Chapter 8
Allergies, Intolerances, and Poisonings from Plant-Based Foods

Margarita Acevedo-Matos, Laura Rincón-Arenas, Stephania Peña-Hernandez, Hugo Corrales-Santander, Marlon Gustavo Múnera Gómez, and Oscar Correa Jiménez

Introduction

Plant-based diets have seen a significant rise globally over the past few decades. An important aspect is that there are various definitions of what these types of diets represent, [1] with perhaps one of the most accepted being the following: "a broad spectrum of dietary patterns that emphasize plant-based products such as fruits and vegetables, whole grains, legumes, nuts and seeds, and alternatives that limit or exclude animal-derived products [2]." With such a generic definition, we

M. Acevedo-Matos
Alergo IPS, Allergy Unit, Pereira, Risaralda, Colombia
e-mail: margarita_acevedomatos@midiagnostica.com

L. Rincón-Arenas
Cayre IPS, Bogotá, D.C., Colombia

S. Peña-Hernandez
La Cardio and HOMI Pediatric Hospital Foundation, Pediatric Gastroenterology Unit, Bogotá, D.C., Colombia
e-mail: spenah@lacardio.org

H. Corrales-Santander
Faculty of Medicine, Pontificia Universidad Javeriana, Bogotá, D.C., Colombia
e-mail: hugocorrales@javeriana.edu.co

M. G. Múnera Gómez
Faculty of Medicine, Universidad Rafael Núñez, Cartagena, Bolívar, Colombia
e-mail: marlon.munera@curnvirtual.edu.co

O. C. Jiménez (✉)
Alergo IPS, Allergy Unit, Pereira, Risaralda, Colombia

Universidad Nacional de Colombia, Faculty of Medicine, Pediatric Pulmonology and Immunology Research Group, Bogotá, D.C., Colombia
e-mail: olcorreaj@unal.edu.co

M. G. Múnera Gómez et al. (eds.), *Allergies, Poisoning and Intolerance to Common Substances*, https://doi.org/10.1007/978-3-031-93658-6_8

increasingly find people following some type of these diets. These dietary trends prevail in both developed and developing countries [3]. Vegetarian or plant-based diets have shown variation in prevalence depending on the geographical area studied, ranging from 4.3% to 30% [4, 5]. Additionally, areas have been documented where the number of vegetarians and vegans has doubled after the COVID pandemic [4].

Various aspects have contributed to the popularity of this type of diet, with perhaps the most important being the health benefits and environmental impact attributed to it [6]. Among these, it has been described that a vegetarian diet helps in the secondary prevention of coronary heart disease by modifying lipid profiles, reducing body mass index, and optimizing serum micronutrient and antioxidant concentrations [7, 8]. Additionally, it has been described that starting a plant-based diet from adolescence is related to a decreased risk of cerebrovascular disease in adulthood [7]. Regarding the environmental impact, it has been documented that vegan and Mediterranean diets present a low carbon footprint, which could represent an effective measure to collectively reduce the environmental impact while improving health [9].

Despite all the noted benefits, like any consumption, plant-based foods also present risks of adverse events. With the rise of these types of diets, it is increasingly common for clinicians to encounter hypersensitivity reactions to these foods, so being familiar with the allergenic nature of these foods is of great importance for appropriate diagnostic and therapeutic approaches. In this same sense, and as happens with reactions to other foods, doctors must keep in mind that both intolerances and poisonings are part of the diagnostic spectrum of reactions or undesirable events associated with the consumption and exposure to plant-based foods [10]. This chapter presents a comprehensive summary of the described plant-based allergens, as well as the main plant-based allergic phenotypes or syndromes. Additionally, it describes issues related to plant-based food intolerances and poisonings.

Plant-Based Allergens

The rapid development of proteomic techniques has enabled the identification, characterization, and expression of recombinant allergens, thereby expanding our understanding of plant-based allergens, their physicochemical characteristics, cross-reactivity, and critical factors for clinical diagnosis. Below is a summary of the generalities of different plant-based allergens by groups of interest:

Fruits

Most fruit allergens belong to the group of plant defense proteins and profilins [11]. They are present in various plant tissues, such as pollen, leaves, roots, seeds, and the fruit itself, with a high degree of structural conservation among different species. This explains the cross-reactivity existing among plant-based allergens [12].

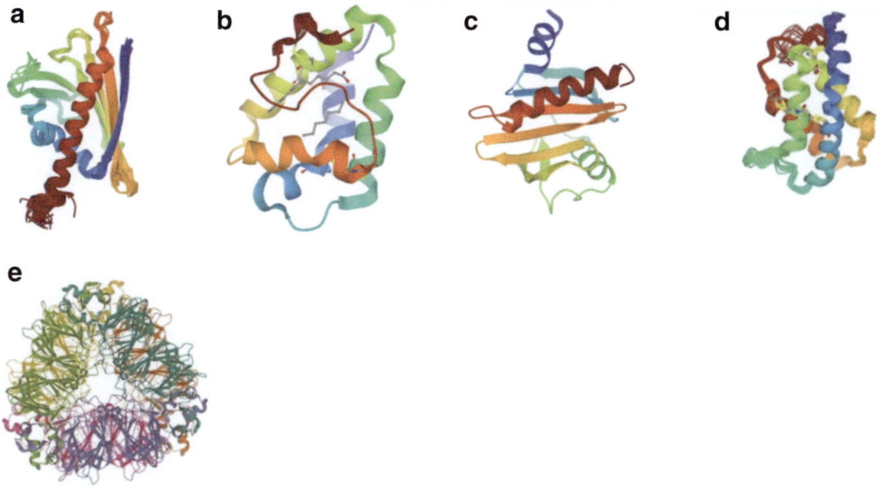

Fig. 8.1 3D structure of allergens reported in several plants. (**a**) birch pollen allergen Bet v 1. (**b**) Pru p3. (**c**) Birch pollen profilin. (**d**) Brazil Nut 2S albumin Ber e 2. (**e**) Structure of seed protein storage 2S albumin

Bet v1 or PR-10 Homologs

These are thermolabile proteins that are sensitive to gastric pH and digestive enzymes. Consequently, initial sensitization occurs via the respiratory tract through birch pollen, and secondarily, symptoms appear upon contact with the oral mucosa with the allergens, found in both the skin and the pulp of the fruit [13, 14]. The Rosaceae family (apple, peach, pear, cherry, apricot, plum, among others) is primarily associated with this syndrome. Birch pollen is the major cause of pollinosis in Northern and Central European countries, with up to 70% of patients allergic to this pollen reporting food allergies (Fig. 8.1) [12].

Lipid Transfer Proteins (LTP)

Lipid transfer proteins (LTP) are small proteins with a rigid tertiary structure formed by four disulfide bridges. Their function is to bind lipids and transfer them between different membrane systems. They are primarily found in the skin and are resistant to hydrolysis by digestive enzymes, mainly gastric pepsin, as well as to thermal hydrolysis and microwave processing [15–17]. These physicochemical properties enable them to directly sensitize through the digestive tract, often causing severe systemic reactions. However, although LTPs are widely distributed in the plant kingdom (Table 8.1), some patients are sensitized only to LTPs from Rosaceae, while others recognize LTPs from other foods and pollens, a condition known as "LTP syndrome." [18].

Table 8.1 List of registered fruit allergens (www.allergen.org March 2023)

Specie	Allergen name	Biochemistry family	Molecular weight (kDa)
Ananas comusus Pineaple	Ana c 1	Profilin	15
	Ana c 2	Bromelin	22.8
Cucumis melo Watermelon	Cuc m 1	Protease	66
	Cuc m 2	Profilin	14
	Cuc m 3	PR-1	16
Actinidia chinensis Golden kiwi	Act c 1	Cistein protease (actinidin)	30
	Act c 5	Kiweline	28
	Act c 8	Homologue of bet v 1	17
	Act c 10	LTP	10
Actinidia deliciosa Green kiwi	Act d 1	Cistein protease (actinidin)	30
	Act d 2	Taumatine	24
	Act d 3		40
	Act d 4	Fitocistatin	11
	Act d 5	Kiwelin	26
	Act d 6	Inhibitor de pectinametilesterase	18
	Act d 7	Pectina metilesterase	50
	Act d 8	Bet v 1 homologue	17
	Act d 9	Profilin	14
	Act d 10	LTP	10
	Act d 11	Bet v 1 homologue	17
	Act d 12	Cupine, 11S globuline	50
	Act d 13	2 s albumine	11
Punica granatum Granade	Pun g 1	LTP	9
	Pun g 2	Gliberitine regulatory protein	7
	Pun g 3	Chitinase III	29
Fragaria ananassa Strawberry	Fra a 1	Bet v 1 homologue	18
	Fra a 3	LTP	9
	Fra a 4	Profilin	13
Malus domestica Apple	Mal d 1	Bet v 1 homologue	17.5
	Mal d 2	Taumatine	23
	Mal d 3	LTP	9
	Mal d 4	Profilin	N.A.
Morus nigra Blackberry	Mor n 3	LTP	10
Prunus armeniaca Apricot	Pru ar 1	Bet v 1 homologue	N.A.
	Pru ar 3	LTP	9
	Pru ar 5	Acidic protein Hev b 5-like	17.4

(continued)

Table 8.1 (continued)

Specie	Allergen name	Biochemistry family	Molecular weight (kDa)
Prunus avium Cherry	Pru av. 1	Bet v 1 homologue	9
	Pru av. 2	Taumatine	23
	Pru av. 3	LTP	10
	Pru av. 4	Profilin	15
	Pru av. 7	Gibberellin regulatory protein	9
Prunus domestica Plum	Pru d 3	LTP	9
Prunus persica Peach	Pru p 1	Bet v 1 homologue	18
	Pru p 2	Taumatine	25–28
	Pru p 3	LTP	10
	Pru p 4	Profilin	14
	Pru p 7	Gibberellin regulatory protein	6910.84 Da (mass spectrometry, mature protein)
	Pru p 9	PR-1	18
	Pru p 10	Poligalacturonidase	46
Pyrus communis Pear	Pyr c 1	Bet v 1 homologue	18
	Pyr c 3	LTP	9
	Pyr c 4	Profilin	14
	Pyr c 5	Isoflavona-reductase	34
Persea americana Avocate	Pers a 1	Endoquitinase	32
Citrus limon Lemon	Cit l 3	LTP	9.6
Citrus reticulata Mandarin	Cit r 3	LTP	9
Citrus sinensis Orange	Cit s 1	Germina	23
	Cit s 2	Profilin	14
	Cit s 3	LTP	9.46
	Cit s 7	Gibberellin regulatory protein	8
Litchi chinensis Lichi	Lit c 1	Profilin	15
Vitis vinífera Grapes	Vit v 1	LTP	9
Musa acuminata Banana	Mus a 1	Profilin	15
	Mus a 2	Quitinase I	33
	Mus a 3	LTP	9
	Mus a 4	Taumatina	20
	Mus a 5	b-1,3 glucanase	30
	Mus a 6	Ascorbato peroxidasae	27

Profilins

Profilins are structurally conserved proteins, with over 70% similarity among them, which accounts for their high cross-reactivity [19–21]. Initial sensitization occurs via the respiratory tract to profilins from pollens, and subsequently to profilins from foods, causing what we know today as "pollen-fruit" syndromes [22, 23]. Similar to Bet v1 homologous proteins, profilins are sensitive to gastric digestion, so these patients present mild symptoms in the oropharyngeal area, [22] although systemic reactions have been described [24].

Chitinases

Chitinases function to degrade fungal walls and the exoskeleton of insects. There is cross-reactivity between the major latex allergen (hevein) and class I chitinases of some fruits, known as the "latex-fruit" syndrome [25]. Fruits implicated in this syndrome include banana, avocado, chestnut, and kiwi [26].

Nuts

The main allergens are storage proteins: cupins (7S globulins or vicilins and 11S globulins or legumins) and prolamins (2S albumins), not only in nut allergies but also in seeds and legumes [27]. These are thermally stable proteins, resistant to proteases, and responsible for severe allergic reactions. Sensitization to Ara h 2 and Ara h 6 (2S albumin) predicts severe reactions to peanuts [28]. Other allergenic proteins of interest include profilins, thaumatin-like proteins, chitinases, oleosins, etc. [29]. (Table 8.2) There is high cross-reactivity between pistachio and cashew, members of the Anacardiaceae family, and between walnut and pecan, members of the Juglandaceae family [30]. Thermal processing can affect allergenicity, as in the case of peanuts, where roasting increases allergenicity and boiling decreases it [31].

Table 8.2 List of registered nut allergens (www.allergen.org March 2023)

Specie	Allergen name	Protein family	Molecular weight (kDa)
Anacardium occidentale Cashew	Ana o 1	Homólogo de vicilina (7S)	50
	Ana o 2	Legumina (11S)	55
	Ana o 3	Albúmina 2S	14
Arachis hypogaea Peanut	Ara h 1	Cupin (Vicillin-type, 7S globulin)	64
	Ara h 2	Conglutin (2S albumin)	17
	Ara h 3	Cupin (Legumin-type, 11S globulin, Glycinin)	60
	Ara h 4	Renamed to Ara h 3.02	15
	Ara h 5	Profilin	15
	Ara h 6	Conglutin (2S albumin)	15
	Ara h 7	Conglutin (2S albumin)	115
	Ara h 8	Pathogenesis-related protein, PR-10, Bet v 1 family member	17
	Ara h 9	Nonspecific lipid-transfer protein type 1	9.8
	Ara h 10	Oleosin	16
	Ara h 11	Oleosin	14
	Ara h 12	Defensin	8 kDa (reducing), 12 kDa (non-reducing), 5.184 kDa (mass)
	Ara h 13	Defensin	8 kDa (reducing), 11 kDa (non-reducing), 5.472 kDa (mass)
	Ara h 14	Oleosin	17.5
	Ara h 15	Oleosin	17
	Ara h 16	Non-specific lipid transfer protein type 2; nsLTP-2	8.5 kDa by SDS PAGE reducing
	Ara h 17	Non-specific lipid transfer protein type 1, nsLTP-1	11 kDa by SDS-PAGE reducing
	Ara h 18	Cyclophilin—peptidyl-prolyl cis-trans isomerase	21
Bertholletia excelsa Brazil nut	Ber e 1	2S sulfur-rich seed storage albumin	9
	Ber e 2	11S globulin seed storage protein	29

(continued)

Table 8.2 (continued)

Specie	Allergen name	Protein family	Molecular weight (kDa)
Castanea sativa Chestnut	Cas s 1	Pathogenesis-related protein, PR-10, Bet v 1 family member	22
	Cas s 5	Chitinase class I	
	Cas s 8	Non-specific lipid transfer protein type 1	12–13 kDa (non-red), 9 kDa (red)
	Cas s 9	Cytosolic class I small heat shock protein; Hsp20	17
Corylus avellana Hazelnut	Cor a 1	Pathogenesis-related protein, PR-10, Bet v 1 family member	17
	Cor a 2	Profilin	14
	Cor a 6	Isoflavone reductase homologue	35
	Cor a 8	Non-specific lipid transfer protein type 1	9
	Cor a 9	11S seed storage globulin (legumin-like)	40
	Cor a 10	Luminal binding protein	70
	Cor a 11	7S seed storage globulin (vicilin-like)	48
	Cor a 12	17 kDa oleosin	17
	Cor a 13	14–16 kDa oleosin	14–16
	Cor a 14	2S albumin	10 kDa reducing
	Cor a 15	Oleosin	17
	Cor a 16	7S globulin seed storage protein (vicilin) containing N-terminal alpha-hairpinin (vicilin_N) peptides	6–8 kDa and 47.5 kDa
Juglans nigra Black walnut	Jug n 1	2S albumin seed storage protein	
	Jug n 2	Vicilin seed storage protein; 7S globulin	
	Jug n 4	Legumin-like seed storage protein; 11S globulin	34 kDa, 22 kDa
Juglans regia English wallnut	Jug r 1	2S albumin seed storage protein	15–16
	Jug r 2	Vicilin (7S globulin) seed storage protein	44
	Jug r 3	Non-specific lipid transfer protein type 1 (nsLTP1)	9
	Jug r 4	11S globulin seed storage protein	58.1
	Jug r 5	PR-10	20
	Jug r 6	7S globulin seed storage protein, vicilin-like protein	47
	Jug r 7	Profilin	13
	Jug r 8	Nonspecific lipid transfer protein type 2; ns-LTP-2	9

(continued)

Table 8.2 (continued)

Specie	Allergen name	Protein family	Molecular weight (kDa)
Pistacia vera Pistachio	Pis v 1	2S albumin	7
	Pis v 2	11S globulin subunit	32
	Pis v 3	Vicillin	55
	Pis v 4	Manganese superoxide dismutase	25.7
	Pis v 5	11S globulin subuni	36
Prunus dulcis Almond	Pru du 1	PR-10, bet v 1-related protein	18
	Pru du 3	Non-specific lipid transfer protein 1 (nsLTP1)	9
	Pru du 4	Profilin	14
	Pru du 5	60 s acidic ribosomal prot. P2	10
	Pru du 6	Amandin, 11S globulin, legumin-like protein	360
	Pru du 8	Antimicrobial seed storage protein	31
	Pru du 10	Mandelonitrile lyase 2; Hydroxynitrile lyase	60

Vegetables

Among vegetable allergens, several proteins have been identified, which we have previously discussed: Bet v 1 homologs, LTPs, and profilins [11, 32]. Distinct allergenic families have been identified compared to those implicated in fruit allergies, such as in the case of potatoes, where a storage protein (patatin) and trypsin inhibitors have been identified [33] (Table 8.3). The main representatives of the Apiaceae family concerning food allergies are celery and carrots.

Table 8.3 List of registered vegetable allergens (www.allergen.org March 2023)

Specie	Allergen name	Protein family	Molecular weight (kDa)
Apium graveolens Celery	Api g 1	Pathogenesis-related protein, PR-10, Bet v 1 family member	16
	Api g 2	Non-specific lipid-transfer protein, type 1	9
	Api g 3	Chlorophyll a-b binding protein, chloroplast	28
	Api g 4	Profilin	14
	Api g 5	FAD-containing oxidase	58
	Api g 6	Non-specific lipid transfer protein type 2	7
	Api g 7	Defensin like protein 1	12
Asparagus officinalis Asparagus	Aspa o 1	Non-specific lipid transfer protein type 1	9
Brassica rapa Field mustard	Bra r 1	2S albumin, napins	10–14
	Bra r 2	Prohevein homologue	25
	Bra r 3	Polcalcin	
Capsicum annuum Bell pepper	Cap a 1	Osmotin-like protein (thaumatin-like protein)	23
	Cap a 1	Profilin	14
	Cap a 1	Gibberellin-regulated protein	10 kDa reducing; 12 kDa non-reducing
Daucus carota Carrot	Dau c 1	Pathogenesis-related protein, PR-10, Bet v 1 family member	16
	Dau c 4	Profilin	14
	Dau c 5	Isoflavone reductase-like protein	33
Lactuca sativa Lettuce	Lac s 1	Non-specific lipid transfer protein	9
Solanum lycopersicum Tomato	Sola L 1	Profilin	14
	Sola L 2	Beta-fructofuranosidase	50
	Sola L 3	Non-specific lipid transfer protein type 1 (nsLTP1)	9
	Sola L 4	Pathogenesis-related protein, PR-10, Bet v 1 family member, TSI-1	20
	Sola L 5	Cyclophilin	19
	Sola L 6	Non-specific lipid transfer protein type 2 (nsLTP2)	7
	Sola L 7	nsLTP type 1	12.5

(continued)

Table 8.3 (continued)

Specie	Allergen name	Protein family	Molecular weight (kDa)
Solanum tuberosum Potato	Sola t 1	Patatin	43
	Sola t 2	Cathepsin D inhibitor PDI	21
	Sola t 3	Cysteine protease inhibitor	21
	Sola t 4	Serine protease inhibitor 7	16
Manihot esculenta Cassava	Man e 5	Glutamic acid rich protein	30
Brassica oleracea Cabbage	Bra o 3	Non-specific lipid transfer protein type 1	9

Table 8.4 List of registered legume allergens (www.allergen.org March 2023)

Specie	Allergen name	Biochemistry family	Molecular weight (kDa)
Lens culinaris Lentil	Len c 1	Gamma-vicilin subunit	47
	Len c 2	Seed-specific biotinylated protein	66
	Len c 3	Nonspecific lipid transfer protein type 1	9
Glycine max Soybean	Gly m 1	Hydrophobic protein from soybean	7
	Gly m 2	Defensin	8
	Gly m 3	Profilin	14
	Gly m 4	Pathogenesis-related protein, PR-10, Bet v 1 family member	17
	Gly m 5	Beta-conglycinin (vicilin, 7S globulin)	
	Gly m 6	Glycinin (legumin, 11S globulin)	
	Gly m 7	Seed biotinylated protein	76.2
	Gly m 8	2S albumin	28
Phaseolus vulgaris Green bean	Pha v 3	Non-specific lipid transfer protein type	9
Lupinus angustifolius Narrow-leaved blu lupin	Lup an 1	Conglutin beta (7S seed storage globulin, vicilin)	55–61
	Lup an 3	Non-specific lipid transfer protein	11
Pisum sativum Pea	Pis s 1	Vicilin	44
	Pis s 1	Convicilin	63
	Pis s 1	nsLTP	9.5

Legumes

Eighty percent of allergenic proteins in legumes correspond to storage globulin proteins, which include vicilins and legumins, while the remaining 20% are components of the albumin fraction, comprising agglutinins, lectins, and protease inhibitors, etc. [34, 35] (Table 8.4). There is a significant identity between the globulins of lentils and peanuts, peas and soybeans, peas and peanuts, chickpeas, peas, and lentils. This similarity is responsible for the cross-reactivity between legumes [36, 37]. Soybean glycinin has a 62% sequence identity with peanut glycinin [38]. There is little cross-reactivity between the vicilins of peanuts and soybeans, but extensive cross-reactivity among lentils, chickpeas, and peas [37, 39].

Soybean allergens depend on the route of sensitization. Thus, inhaled allergens involve proteins from the husk, Gly m 1 and Gly m 2, typically presenting as asthma as part of occupational allergy, while digestive allergens Gly m 5 and Gly m 6 are associated with severe reactions [40, 41]. Most legumes are consumed after thermal processing, whether boiled, roasted, or fried, which can alter their allergenicity [42, 43].

Cereals and Seeds

The consumption of seeds has increased in recent years due to their nutritional benefits, and although they share the same biological function, they belong to different botanical families with no taxonomic relationship between them. In the case of cereals, they belong to the grass family (except for buckwheat or Sarraceno wheat). They are consumed as grains, ground, oils, pasta, beverages, and as condiments or thickeners in sauces and dressings. Our review considers yellow mustard, sesame, and wheat. Cereal proteins are classified according to their solubility: in water (albumins), saline solutions (globulins), alcohol (prolamins), and acidic and alkaline solutions (glutenins) (Table 8.5). Gluten makes up 80% of grain proteins and is composed of gliadins and glutenins, responsible for food allergies [44]. There is a phenotype of wheat-dependent, exercise-induced anaphylaxis, where the responsible allergen in most cases is ω-5 gliadin (Tri a 19) [45]. Sensitization can also be through inhalation, generally as occupational asthma, called "baker's asthma," with the main sensitization to α-amylase/trypsin inhibitors [46].

Table 8.5 List of registered cereal and seed allergens (www.allergen.org March 2023)

Specie	Allergen name	Protein family	Molecular weight (kDa)
Sinapsis alba Yellow mustard	Sin a 1	2S albumin	14
	Sin a 2	11S globulin (legumin-like) seed storage protein	51
	Sin a 3	Non-specific lipid transfer protein type 1	12.3
	Sin a 3	Profilin	13/14
Sesamum indicum Sesame	Ses i 1	2S albumin	9
	Ses i 2	2S albumin	7
	Ses i 3	7S vicilin-like globulin	45
	Ses i 4	Oleosin	17
	Ses i 5	Oleosin	15
	Ses i 6	11S globulin	52
	Ses i 7	11S globulin	57

(continued)

Table 8.5 (continued)

Specie	Allergen name	Protein family	Molecular weight (kDa)
Triticum aestivum Wheat	Tri a 12	Profilin	14
	Tri a 14	Non-specific lipid transfer protein 1	9
	Tri a 15	Monomeric alpha-amylase inhibitor 0.28	
	Tri a 17	Beta-amylase	56
	Tri a 18	Agglutinin isolectin 1	
	Tri a 19	Omega-5 gliadin, seed storage protein	65
	Tri a 20	Gamma gliadin	35–38
	Tri a 21	Alpha-beta-gliadin	
	Tri a 25	Thioredoxin	
	Tri a 26	High molecular weight glutenin	88
	Tri a 27	Thiol reductase homologue	27
	Tri a 28	Dimeric alpha-amylase inhibitor 0.19	13
	Tri a 29	Tetrameric alpha-amylase inhibitor CM1/CM2	13
	Tri a 30	Tetrameric alpha-amylase inhibitor CM3	16
	Tri a 31	Triosephosphate-isomerase	
	Tri a 32	1-cys-peroxiredoxin	
	Tri a 33	Serpin	
	Tri a 34	Glyceraldehyde-3-phosphate-dehydrogenase	
	Tri a 35	Dehydrin	
	Tri a 36	Low molecular weight glutenin GluB3–23	40
	Tri a 37	Alpha purothionin	12
	Tri a 39	Serine protease inhibitor-like protein	
	Tri a 40	Chloroform/methanol-soluble (CM) 17 protein [alpha-amylase inhibitor]	15.96
	Tri a 41	Mitochondrial ubiquitin ligase activator of NFKB 1	
	Tri a 42	Hypothetical protein from cDNA	
	Tri a 43	Hypothetical protein from cDNA	
	Tri a 44	Endosperm transfer cell specific PR60 precursor	
	Tri a 45	Elongation factor 1 (EIF1)	

Cannabis

Cannabis sativa is a plant belonging to the Cannabaceae family. It is the most widely used illicit drug in the world, and in the last decade, its use has expanded in the form of hemp seeds, marijuana leaves or flowers, hashish (dried resin), and medicinal drugs. Can s 3 (LTP) is the major allergen and a marker of severe reactions [47–49] (Table 8.6). There have also been cases of occupational allergy, with respiratory manifestations (rhinitis and asthma), urticaria and angioedema, and contact dermatitis [50].

Table 8.6 List of registered allergens of *Cannabis sativa* (www.allergen.org March 2023)

Specie	Allergen name	Protein family	Molecular weight (kDa)
Cannabis sativa Indian hemp	Can s 2	Profilin	14
	Can s 3	Non-specific lipid transfer protein type 1	9
	Can s 4	Oxygen evolving enhancer protein 2	27.3
	Can s 5	Pathogenesis-related protein PR-10, Bet v 1-related protein	17.7

Table 8.7 Prevalent clinical syndromes in vegetable allergy

	Oral allergy syndrome	LTP syndrome	Latex-fruit syndrome	Systemic reactions
Implicated proteins	PR-10 or Bet v1 homologs Profilins	LTP (Lipid Transfer Proteins)	Chitinases	ω-5-gliadin LTP Storage proteins from seeds
Properties of the implicated proteins	Sensitive to cooking and digestion	Resistant to cooking and digestion	Resistant to digestion	Resistant to cooking and digestion
Symptoms	Oral pruritus, ear pruritus, lip and perioral erythema, lip and glottis edema	Anaphylaxis	Urticaria, anaphylaxis	Anaphylaxis with or without the involvement of cofactors Exercise-induced anaphylaxis
Commonly implicated vegetables	Melon, watermelon, apple, hazelnut, carrot, celery	Rosaceae, nuts, lettuce, tomato	Latex, banana, chestnut, kiwi, avocado	Wheat, nuts

Phenotypes of Food Allergy of Plant Origin

The pattern of sensitization to different allergens depends on the geographic area. Sensitization to Bet v 1 homologs is significantly high in northern and central European countries with exposure to tree pollen from the Fagaceae and Betulaceae families [51]. While in the Mediterranean area, the relevant allergens are profilin and LTP sensitization. This distribution and the physicochemical characteristics of the different allergenic proteins determine the clinical manifestations [52]. Below, we describe the main phenotypes or allergic syndromes associated with plant-based sources (Table 8.7).

Oral Allergy Syndrome

Oral allergy syndrome is characterized by local symptoms immediately after contact of the oral mucosa with the plant, often including oral and ear itching, lip and perioral erythema, and even lip and glottis edema. This is since the sensitizing allergens are labile pollen proteins, such as Bet v 1 homologs and profilins, although it has also been observed in subjects not sensitized to pollen [14, 53], as well as systemic reactions [54]. Sensitization can be evaluated with pollen SPT, prick-to-prick with fresh food, and available in vitro recombinants. ImmunoCAP specific IgE (Thermo Fischer Scientific) includes Phl p 12, Bet v 2, Pru p 4, and Hev b 8, four profilins from grass pollen, birch pollen, peach, and latex, and for PR-10, Bet v 1 is available. This association has been described not only between pollen and fruits but also between pollen and nuts, such as Artemisia pollen and fruits like hazelnut, sunflower seeds, pistachio, almond, and peanut [55, 56], and parietaria pollen and pistachio [57], pollen and vegetables like birch pollen, celery, and carrot [58]. Oral allergy syndrome has also been described with the ingestion of mustard and sesame [59, 60]. Since in most cases the symptoms are mild, no special management measures are required. Some studies have shown that after pollen immunotherapy in patients with respiratory symptoms, the resolution of oral symptoms with vegetable intake was demonstrated in subjects sensitized to profilins and Bet v 1 [61, 62].

LTP Syndrome

As we explained earlier, in the Mediterranean area, lipid transfer proteins (LTPs) are the most relevant allergens, often causing systemic involvement without the need for associated pollinosis, with or without cofactors [16, 63, 64]. The profile of these patients is heterogeneous, with some patients sensitized only to LTPs from rosaceae (peach, apple, plum, pear), others recognizing LTPs from other foods (kiwi, tomato, lettuce, mustard, walnut, hazelnut, peanut), and even pollens, which has been termed "LTP syndrome" [65]. Pru p 3 is the main allergen of peach and the first LTP identified and characterized, found mainly in the skin. Barber et al. in Spain described that approximately 2% of adults and 4% of children are sensitized to Pru p 3, of which 50% report food allergy [66]. The severity of clinical symptoms varies from contact urticaria to anaphylaxis, but systemic reactions are common in any case [63]. A frequent characteristic of these reactions is the requirement of a cofactor (NSAIDs, exercise, and alcohol) [64, 67].

Latex-Fruit Syndrome

Chitinases are the allergen responsible for the cross-reactivity between latex and certain fruits such as banana, avocado, chestnut, and kiwi [25]. An association between latex allergy and other plant foods such as papaya, tomato, pineapple, passion fruit, mango, and pineapple has also been described. These proteins are stable to digestion, which explains systemic reactions as the main clinical manifestation, with anaphylaxis occurring in 42% of cases [26].

Systemic Reactions

Different proteins can cause systemic reactions after the ingestion of vegetables, with or without the involvement of cofactors. Cardona et al. reported 74 cases of anaphylaxis in the presence of cofactors, where 99% of the foods were of plant origin, and the main allergen was LTP. In 58% of cases, the cofactor was NSAIDs, in 52.7% exercise, and 12.2% alcohol [68]. Wheat-dependent, exercise-induced anaphylaxis, with ω-5-gliadin as the main allergen, followed by wheat LTP (Tri a 14) [69, 70], has become a challenge in allergy consultations. It depends on the intensity of exercise, the amount of allergen ingested, and the interval between ingestion and the onset of symptoms, which can be up to 4 h, and patients do not have a history of cereal allergy in childhood [70].

Nut allergy, especially peanut, is one of the most frequent causes of anaphylaxis [55], particularly in patients with multiple food allergies [71] and in patients without pollen allergy [72]. Storage proteins, especially 2S albumin, are stable to cooking and digestion [73]; consequently, approximately 90% of patients sensitized to Ara h 2 experience severe reactions to peanuts [74].

Intolerance to Foods of Plant Origin

Nonallergic food hypersensitivity or nonallergic food reactions are more common than food allergies and fall under non-immune-mediated adverse food reactions; unlike allergic reactions, the severity of symptoms depends directly on the amount of food ingested [75, 76].

Food intolerances or non-immunological adverse reactions to food can be divided into those that are independent of the host and those dependent on the host. Among the most common host-dependent adverse reactions is lactose intolerance; however, there are intolerances to other carbohydrates found in foods such as fruits, vegetables, or honey, like fructose. Fructose intolerance has a clinical presentation similar to lactose intolerance, but its mechanism is unclear since studies have not shown a difference in the expression of the GLUT5 transporter in intolerant versus tolerant patients. Clinically, patients manifest with osmotic diarrhea due to undigested fructose in the intestinal lumen, causing bacterial fermentation at the colonic level. Diagnosis can be made through a hydrogen breath test following a fructose load. Management of fructose malabsorption is based on daily intakes of fructose less than 10 g/day [77].

Fermentable oligosaccharides, disaccharides, monosaccharides, and polyols (FODMAPs) are another group of natural carbohydrates found in a wide variety of foods, related to irritable bowel syndrome (IBS). The osmotic effect generated by carbohydrate malabsorption increases water content in the intestinal lumen, accelerates intestinal transit, and consequently fermented by colonic bacteria, producing gas associated with bloating and abdominal pain [78]. Therapy involves an exclusion diet of FODMAP-containing foods, adapted by a nutritionist, considering that the tolerance threshold may differ among patients [77].

Other components may be added to or naturally found in some foods, such as salicylates, causing intolerances. Vegetables containing salicylates include asparagus, soy, beetroot, broccoli, Brussels sprouts, bok choy, bell pepper, cauliflower, eggplant, endive, fennel, leek, cabbage, cucumber, lettuce, mushroom, onion, arugula, radish, spinach, tomato, and zucchini; beetroot has the highest salicylate content at 26.93 mg/kg versus soy with the lowest at 1.28 mg/kg. Lastly, histamine is a biogenic amine produced and degraded in the human body and found in numerous foods, such as eggplant, avocado, spinach, and tomatoes [79]. Symptoms of histamine intolerance are nonspecific and may have digestive and extra-digestive manifestations, occurring during or just after ingestion. Symptoms result from accumulated ingested histamine and the inability to degrade it due to low levels of diamine oxidase, the enzyme involved in histamine metabolism. The approach should exclude food allergies, celiac disease, and inflammatory bowel disease, and a food diary should establish a causal relationship between food intake and symptom onset, with improvement following a low-histamine diet. Therapy includes antihistamines, diamine oxidase supplements, and low-histamine diets [80].

Food Poisoning Associated with Vegetables

Foodborne illnesses not mediated by allergic or intolerance reactions are classified into two types: (a) infections, which occur when a pathogen is ingested with food, establishes itself, and multiplies in humans, and (b) intoxications, which occur when a pathogen establishes itself in a food product, produces, and releases toxins, which are then ingested by humans [81].

Vegetables provide an environment where a wide variety of microorganisms can develop and can contain many contaminants of biological or chemical origin; these include viruses, bacteria, parasites, chemicals, toxins, and allergens that cause a wide range of conditions [82, 83]. These are responsible for both acute and chronic infections and intoxications, with high associated morbidity and mortality that significantly increase direct and indirect health costs. Although they more frequently affect developing countries and the child population, they are considered a global public health problem because increasing international trade raises the risk of contamination in exported foods. Additionally, migration and travel can expose populations to new hazards [82, 84]. The global burden generated is comparable to that of major infectious diseases, HIV/AIDS, malaria, and tuberculosis [82]. Much of this is preventable; therefore, there is an urgent need to develop cost-effective food hygiene interventions that can be implemented in resource-poor settings [82].

Clinical manifestations are variable, ranging from diarrhea, vomiting, and abdominal pain to others like meningitis, septicemia, hemorrhagic colitis, hemolytic uremic syndrome, autoimmune complications, and some types of cancer [84, 85]. Intervention measures will be according to the type of manifestation presented and are mostly supportive.

Conclusions and Future Directions

Fruits and vegetables are an important source of allergens associated with different syndromic conditions of clinical relevance in allergy practice. However, clinicians must also consider other causes of reactions or adverse events associated with plant-based foods: intolerances and intoxications, which are often more frequent and have clinical presentations that guide appropriate diagnosis. An adequate approach to these cases leads to less stress associated with uncertainty about the nature of the reactions the patient presents. Although the consumption of vegetables has increased considerably, we still lack epidemiological characterization of allergic reactions, intolerances, and intoxications from such consumption. Therefore, in the medium term, efforts should be made to better understand the epidemiological dynamics and mechanisms involved.

Glossary

Glossary of Acronyms

FODMAPs Fermentable Oligosaccharides, Disaccharides, Monosaccharides, and Polyols
GLUT5 Glucose Transporter 5
HMW High Molecular Weight
IBS Irritable Bowel Syndrome
IgE Immunoglobulin E
LTP Lipid Transfer Protein
PR-10 Pathogenesis-Related Protein 10
SIAIP Italian Society for Pediatric Allergy and Immunology
SIGENP Italian Society for Pediatric Gastroenterology, Hepatology, and Nutrition
SPT Skin Prick Test

Glossary of Terms

Allergens Substances that can cause an allergic reaction.
Anaphylaxis A severe, potentially life-threatening allergic reaction.
Celiac Disease An autoimmune disorder where ingestion of gluten leads to damage in the small intestine.
Cross-reactivity When the immune system reacts to similar proteins in different substances.
Dermatitis Inflammation of the skin.
Eczema Condition that makes the skin red and itchy.

Food Allergy An immune system reaction that occurs soon after eating a certain food.

Food Intolerance Difficulty in digesting certain foods.

Gluten A group of proteins found in wheat and related grains.

Histamine A compound involved in local immune responses and regulating physiological functions in the gut.

Hypersensitivity Excessive or inappropriate response of the immune system to a substance.

Immune System The body's defense against infectious organisms and other invaders.

Immunoglobulin E (IgE) A class of antibodies produced by the immune system.

Lactose Intolerance The inability to digest lactose, a sugar found in milk and dairy products.

Pathogen A bacterium, virus, or other microorganism that can cause disease.

Proteins Large biomolecules consisting of one or more long chains of amino acid residues.

Sensitization The process by which exposure to an allergen causes an allergic reaction.

Symptoms A physical or mental feature indicating a condition of disease.

Toxins Poisonous substances produced within living cells or organisms.

Urticaria (Hives) A skin rash triggered by a reaction to food, medicine, or other irritants.

References

1. Klapp AL, Feil N, Risius A. A global analysis of National Dietary Guidelines on plant-based diets and substitutions for animal-based foods. Curr Dev Nutr. 2022;6(11):nzac144.
2. Kent G, Kehoe L, Flynn A, Walton J. Plant-based diets: a review of the definitions and nutritional role in the adult diet. Proc Nutr Soc. 2022;81(1):62–74.
3. Dorgbetor IK, Ondrasek G, Kutnjak H, Mikuš O. What if the world went vegan? A review of the impact on natural resources, climate change, and economies. Agriculture. 2022;12(10):1518.
4. Al-Mohaithef M. Prevalence of vegan/vegetarian diet and eating behavior among Saudi adults and its correlation with body mass index: a cross-sectional study. Front Nutr. 2022;9:966629.
5. Agrawal S, Millett CJ, Dhillon PK, Subramanian SV, Ebrahim S. Type of vegetarian diet, obesity and diabetes in adult Indian population. Nutr J. 2014;13:89.
6. Key TJ, Papier K, Tong TYN. Plant-based diets and long-term health: findings from the EPIC-Oxford study. Proc Nutr Soc. 2022;81(2):190–8.
7. Babalola F, Adesuyi A, David F, Kolajo BA, Urhi A, Akinade O, et al. A comprehensive review on the effects of vegetarian diets on coronary heart disease. Cureus. 2022;14(10):e29843.
8. Koutentakis M, Surma S, Rogula S, Filipiak KJ, Gasecka A. The effect of a vegan diet on the cardiovascular system. J Cardiovasc Dev Dis. 2023;10(3):94.
9. Dixon KA, Michelsen MK, Carpenter CL. Modern diets and the health of our planet: an investigation into the environmental impacts of food choices. Nutrients. 2023;15(3):692.
10. Patel P, Komorowski AS, Mack DP. An allergist's approach to food poisoning. Ann Allergy Asthma Immunol. 2023;130(4):444–51.
11. Breiteneder H, Ebner C. Molecular and biochemical classification of plant-derived food allergens. J Allergy Clin Immunol. 2000;106(1 Pt 1):27–36.

12. Jenkins JA, Griffiths-Jones S, Shewry PR, Breiteneder H, Mills EN. Structural relatedness of plant food allergens with specific reference to cross-reactive allergens: an in silico analysis. J Allergy Clin Immunol. 2005;115(1):163–70.
13. Aalberse RC. Structural biology of allergens. J Allergy Clin Immunol. 2000;106(2):228–38.
14. Kazemi-Shirazi L, Pauli G, Purohit A, Spitzauer S, Froschl R, Hoffmann-Sommergruber K, et al. Quantitative IgE inhibition experiments with purified recombinant allergens indicate pollen-derived allergens as the sensitizing agents responsible for many forms of plant food allergy. J Allergy Clin Immunol. 2000;105(1 Pt 1):116–25.
15. Asero R, Mistrello G, Roncarolo D, de Vries SC, Gautier MF, Ciurana CL, et al. Lipid transfer protein: a pan-allergen in plant-derived foods that is highly resistant to pepsin digestion. Int Arch Allergy Immunol. 2000;122(1):20–32.
16. Pastorello EA, Pompei C, Pravettoni V, Farioli L, Calamari AM, Scibilia J, et al. Lipid-transfer protein is the major maize allergen maintaining IgE-binding activity after cooking at 100 degrees C, as demonstrated in anaphylactic patients and patients with positive double-blind, placebo-controlled food challenge results. J Allergy Clin Immunol. 2003;112(4):775–83.
17. Garino C, Zitelli F, Travaglia F, Colsson JD, Cravotto G, Arlorio M. Evaluation of the impact of sequential microwave/ultrasound processing on the IgE binding properties of Pru p 3 in treated peach juice. J Agric Food Chem. 2012;60(35):8755–62.
18. Diaz-Perales A, Lombardero M, Sanchez-Monge R, Garcia-Selles FJ, Pernas M, Fernandez-Rivas M, et al. Lipid-transfer proteins as potential plant panallergens: cross-reactivity among proteins of Artemisia pollen, Castanea nut and Rosaceae fruits, with different IgE-binding capacities. Clin Exp Allergy. 2000;30(10):1403–10.
19. Rodriguez-Perez R, Fernandez-Rivas M, Gonzalez-Mancebo E, Sanchez-Monge R, Diaz-Perales A, Salcedo G. Peach profilin: cloning, heterologous expression and cross-reactivity with Bet v 2. Allergy. 2003;58(7):635–40.
20. Sirvent S, Tordesillas L, Villalba M, Diaz-Perales A, Cuesta-Herranz J, Salcedo G, et al. Pollen and plant food profilin allergens show equivalent IgE reactivity. Ann Allergy Asthma Immunol. 2011;106(5):429–35.
21. Radauer C, Willerroider M, Fuchs H, Hoffmann-Sommergruber K, Thalhamer J, Ferreira F, et al. Cross-reactive and species-specific immunoglobulin E epitopes of plant profilins: an experimental and structure-based analysis. Clin Exp Allergy. 2006;36(7):920–9.
22. Santos A, Van Ree R. Profilins: mimickers of allergy or relevant allergens? Int Arch Allergy Immunol. 2011;155(3):191–204.
23. Ganglberger E, Radauer C, Wagner S, Riordain G, Beezhold DH, Brehler R, et al. Hev b 8, the Hevea brasiliensis latex profilin, is a cross-reactive allergen of latex, plant foods and pollen. Int Arch Allergy Immunol. 2001;125(3):216–27.
24. Fah J, Wuthrich B, Vieths S. Anaphylactic reaction to lychee fruit: evidence for sensitization to profilin. Clin Exp Allergy. 1995;25(10):1018–23.
25. Radauer C, Adhami F, Furtler I, Wagner S, Allwardt D, Scala E, et al. Latex-allergic patients sensitized to the major allergen hevein and hevein-like domains of class I chitinases show no increased frequency of latex-associated plant food allergy. Mol Immunol. 2011;48(4):600–9.
26. Blanco C. Latex-fruit syndrome. Curr Allergy Asthma Rep. 2003;3(1):47–53.
27. Smeekens JM, Bagley K, Kulis M. Tree nut allergies: allergen homology, cross-reactivity, and implications for therapy. Clin Exp Allergy. 2018;48(7):762–72.
28. Kukkonen AK, Pelkonen AS, Makinen-Kiljunen S, Voutilainen H, Makela MJ. Ara h 2 and Ara 6 are the best predictors of severe peanut allergy: a double-blind placebo-controlled study. Allergy. 2015;70(10):1239–45.
29. Shreffler WG, Castro RR, Kucuk ZY, Charlop-Powers Z, Grishina G, Yoo S, et al. The major glycoprotein allergen from Arachis hypogaea, Ara h 1, is a ligand of dendritic cell-specific ICAM-grabbing nonintegrin and acts as a Th2 adjuvant in vitro. J Immunol. 2006;177(6):3677–85.
30. Kuzminski A, Przybyszewski M, Przybyszewska J, Ukleja-Sokolowska N, Palgan K, Bartuzi Z. Tree nut allergy. Postepy Dermatol Alergol. 2021;38(4):544–9.
31. Palladino C, Breiteneder H. Peanut allergens. Mol Immunol. 2018;100:58–70.

32. Scheurer S, Wangorsch A, Haustein D, Vieths S. Cloning of the minor allergen Api g 4 profilin from celery (Apium graveolens) and its cross-reactivity with birch pollen profilin Bet v 2. Clin Exp Allergy. 2000;30(7):962–71.
33. Schmidt MHH, Raulf-Heimsoth M, Posch A. Evaluation of patatin as a major cross-reactive allergen in latex-induced potato allergy. Ann Allergy Asthma Immunol. 2002;89(6):613–8.
34. Verma AK, Kumar S, Das M, Dwivedi PD. A comprehensive review of legume allergy. Clin Rev Allergy Immunol. 2013;45(1):30–46.
35. Sanchez-Monge R, Pascual CY, Diaz-Perales A, Fernandez-Crespo J, Martin-Esteban M, Salcedo G. Isolation and characterization of relevant allergens from boiled lentils. J Allergy Clin Immunol. 2000;106(5):955–61.
36. Lopez-Torrejon G, Salcedo G, Martin-Esteban M, Diaz-Perales A, Pascual CY, Sanchez-Monge R. Len c 1, a major allergen and vicilin from lentil seeds: protein isolation and cDNA cloning. J Allergy Clin Immunol. 2003;112(6):1208–15.
37. Wensing M, Knulst AC, Piersma S, O'Kane F, Knol EF, Koppelman SJ. Patients with anaphylaxis to pea can have peanut allergy caused by cross-reactive IgE to vicilin (Ara h 1). J Allergy Clin Immunol. 2003;111(2):420–4.
38. Barre A, Jacquet G, Sordet C, Culerrier R, Rouge P. Homology modelling and conformational analysis of IgE-binding epitopes of Ara h 3 and other legumin allergens with a cupin fold from tree nuts. Mol Immunol. 2007;44(12):3243–55.
39. Beardslee TA, Zeece MG, Sarath G, Markwell JP. Soybean glycinin G1 acidic chain shares IgE epitopes with peanut allergen Ara h 3. Int Arch Allergy Immunol. 2000;123(4):299–307.
40. Ebisawa M, Brostedt P, Sjolander S, Sato S, Borres MP, Ito K. Gly m 2S albumin is a major allergen with a high diagnostic value in soybean-allergic children. J Allergy Clin Immunol. 2013;132(4):976–8 e1-5.
41. Berneder M, Bublin M, Hoffmann-Sommergruber K, Hawranek T, Lang R. Allergen chip diagnosis for soy-allergic patients: Gly m 4 as a marker for severe food-allergic reactions to soy. Int Arch Allergy Immunol. 2013;161(3):229–33.
42. Verma AK, Kumar S, Das M, Dwivedi PD. Impact of thermal processing on legume allergens. Plant Foods Hum Nutr. 2012;67(4):430–41.
43. Rodriguez-Mazariego ME, Fuentes Aparicio V, Bartolome Zavala B, Acevedo Matos M, Zapatero RL. Broad bean-induced anaphylaxis: a case report. J Investig Allergol Clin Immunol. 2016;26(6):374–5.
44. Jin Y, Acharya HG, Acharya D, Jorgensen R, Gao H, Secord J, et al. Advances in molecular mechanisms of wheat Allergenicity in animal models: a comprehensive review. Molecules. 2019;24(6):1142.
45. Morita E, Matsuo H, Chinuki Y, Takahashi H, Dahlstrom J, Tanaka A. Food-dependent exercise-induced anaphylaxis -importance of omega-5 gliadin and HMW-glutenin as causative antigens for wheat-dependent exercise-induced anaphylaxis. Allergol Int. 2009;58(4):493–8.
46. Quirce S, Diaz-Perales A. Diagnosis and management of grain-induced asthma. Allergy Asthma Immunol Res. 2013;5(6):348–56.
47. Decuyper II, Van Gasse AL, Faber MA, Elst J, Mertens C, Rihs HP, et al. Exploring the diagnosis and profile of cannabis allergy. J Allergy Clin Immunol Pract. 2019;7(3):983–9 e5.
48. Alkhammash S, Tsui H, Thomson DMP. Cannabis and hemp seed allergy. J Allergy Clin Immunol Pract. 2019;7(7):2429–30 e1.
49. Gamboa P, Sanchez-Monge R, Sanz ML, Palacin A, Salcedo G, Diaz-Perales A. Sensitization to Cannabis sativa caused by a novel allergenic lipid transfer protein, Can s 3. J Allergy Clin Immunol. 2007;120(6):1459–60.
50. Decuyper II, Green BJ, Sussman GL, Ebo DG, Silvers WS, Pacheco K, et al. Occupational allergies to cannabis. J Allergy Clin Immunol Pract. 2020;8(10):3331–8.
51. Hauser M, Asam C, Himly M, Palazzo P, Voltolini S, Montanari C, et al. Bet v 1-like pollen allergens of multiple Fagales species can sensitize atopic individuals. Clin Exp Allergy. 2011;41(12):1804–14.

52. Fernandez-Rivas M, Bolhaar S, Gonzalez-Mancebo E, Asero R, van Leeuwen A, Bohle B, et al. Apple allergy across Europe: how allergen sensitization profiles determine the clinical expression of allergies to plant foods. J Allergy Clin Immunol. 2006;118(2):481–8.
53. Asero R, Mistrello G, Roncarolo D, Amato S, Zanoni D, Barocci F, et al. Detection of clinical markers of sensitization to profilin in patients allergic to plant-derived foods. J Allergy Clin Immunol. 2003;112(2):427–32.
54. Gomez Torrijos E, Gratacos Gomez AR, Gonzalez Jimenez OM, Joyanes Romo JB, Palacios Canas A, Garcia Rodriguez R. Profilins and food-dependent exercise-induced anaphylaxis. J Investig Allergol Clin Immunol. 2021;31(4):349–50.
55. Du Toit G, Lack G. Optimizing the diagnosis of peanut and tree nut allergy. Clin Exp Allergy. 2003;33(8):1019–22.
56. Garcia Ortiz JC, Cosmes PM, Lopez-Asunsolo A. Allergy to foods in patients monosensitized to Artemisia pollen. Allergy. 1996;51(12):927–31.
57. Liccardi G, Russo M, Mistrello G, Falagiani P, D'Amato M, D'Amato G. Sensitization to pistachio is common in Parietaria allergy. Allergy. 1999;54(6):643–5.
58. Lopez-Matas MA, Ferrer A, Larramendi CH, Huertas AJ, Pagan JA, Garcia-Abujeta JL, et al. In vitro cross-reactivity between tomato and other plant allergens. Ann Allergy Asthma Immunol. 2009;103(5):425–31.
59. Dalal I, Goldberg M, Katz Y. Sesame seed food allergy. Curr Allergy Asthma Rep. 2012;12(4):339–45.
60. Vereda A, Sirvent S, Villalba M, Rodriguez R, Cuesta-Herranz J, Palomares O. Improvement of mustard (Sinapis alba) allergy diagnosis and management by linking clinical features and component-resolved approaches. J Allergy Clin Immunol. 2011;127(5):1304–7.
61. Asero R. Fennel, cucumber, and melon allergy successfully treated with pollen-specific injection immunotherapy. Ann Allergy Asthma Immunol. 2000;84(4):460–2.
62. Nothegger B, Reider N, Covaciu CE, Cova V, Ahammer L, Eidelpes R, et al. Oral birch pollen immunotherapy with apples: results of a phase II clinical pilot study. Immun Inflamm Dis. 2021;9(2):503–11.
63. Pascal M, Munoz-Cano R, Reina Z, Palacin A, Vilella R, Picado C, et al. Lipid transfer protein syndrome: clinical pattern, cofactor effect and profile of molecular sensitization to plant-foods and pollens. Clin Exp Allergy. 2012;42(10):1529–39.
64. Romano A, Scala E, Rumi G, Gaeta F, Caruso C, Alonzi C, et al. Lipid transfer proteins: the most frequent sensitizer in Italian subjects with food-dependent exercise-induced anaphylaxis. Clin Exp Allergy. 2012;42(11):1643–53.
65. Garcia-Selles FJ, Diaz-Perales A, Sanchez-Monge R, Alcantara M, Lombardero M, Barber D, et al. Patterns of reactivity to lipid transfer proteins of plant foods and Artemisia pollen: an in vivo study. Int Arch Allergy Immunol. 2002;128(2):115–22.
66. Barber D, de la Torre F, Feo F, Florido F, Guardia P, Moreno C, et al. Understanding patient sensitization profiles in complex pollen areas: a molecular epidemiological study. Allergy. 2008;63(11):1550–8.
67. Skypala IJ, Bartra J, Ebo DG, Antje Faber M, Fernandez-Rivas M, Gomez F, et al. The diagnosis and management of allergic reactions in patients sensitized to non-specific lipid transfer proteins. Allergy. 2021;76(8):2433–46.
68. Cardona V, Luengo O, Garriga T, Labrador-Horrillo M, Sala-Cunill A, Izquierdo A, et al. Co-factor-enhanced food allergy. Allergy. 2012;67(10):1316–8.
69. Pastorello EA, Farioli L, Stafylaraki C, Scibilia J, Mirone C, Pravettoni V, et al. Wheat-dependent exercise-induced anaphylaxis caused by a lipid transfer protein and not by omega-5 gliadin. Ann Allergy Asthma Immunol. 2014;112(4):386–7 e1.
70. Palosuo K. Update on wheat hypersensitivity. Curr Opin Allergy Clin Immunol. 2003;3(3):205–9.
71. Sicherer SH, Furlong TJ, DeSimone J, Sampson HA. Self-reported allergic reactions to peanut on commercial airliners. J Allergy Clin Immunol. 1999;104(1):186–9.

72. Schocker F, Luttkopf D, Muller U, Thomas P, Vieths S, Becker WM. IgE binding to unique hazelnut allergens: identification of non pollen-related and heat-stable hazelnut allergens eliciting severe allergic reactions. Eur J Nutr. 2000;39(4):172–80.
73. Verhoeckx KCM, Vissers YM, Baumert JL, Faludi R, Feys M, Flanagan S, et al. Food processing and allergenicity. Food Chem Toxicol. 2015;80:223–40.
74. Klemans RJ, van Os-Medendorp H, Blankestijn M, Bruijnzeel-Koomen CA, Knol EF, Knulst AC. Diagnostic accuracy of specific IgE to components in diagnosing peanut allergy: a systematic review. Clin Exp Allergy. 2015;45(4):720–30.
75. Turnbull JL, Adams HN, Gorard DA. Review article: the diagnosis and management of food allergy and food intolerances. Aliment Pharmacol Ther. 2015;41(1):3–25.
76. Gargano D, Appanna R, Santonicola A, De Bartolomeis F, Stellato C, Cianferoni A, et al. Food allergy and intolerance: a narrative review on nutritional concerns. Nutrients. 2021;13(5):1638.
77. Berni Canani R, Caffarelli C, Calvani M, Martelli A, Carucci L, Cozzolino T, et al. Diagnostic therapeutic care pathway for pediatric food allergies and intolerances in Italy: a joint position paper by the Italian Society for Pediatric Gastroenterology Hepatology and Nutrition (SIGENP) and the Italian Society for Pediatric Allergy and Immunology (SIAIP). Ital J Pediatr. 2022;48(1):87.
78. Muthukumar J, Selvasekaran P, Lokanadham M, Chidambaram R. Food and food products associated with food allergy and food intolerance – an overview. Food Res Int. 2020;138(Pt B):109780.
79. Tuck CJ, Biesiekierski JR, Schmid-Grendelmeier P, Pohl D. Food intolerances. Nutrients. 2019;11:7.
80. Shulpekova YO, Nechaev VM, Popova IR, Deeva TA, Kopylov AT, Malsagova KA, et al. Food intolerance: the role of histamine. Nutrients. 2021;13(9):3207.
81. Bintsis T. Foodborne pathogens. AIMS Microbiol. 2017;3(3):529–63.
82. Havelaar AH, Kirk MD, Torgerson PR, Gibb HJ, Hald T, Lake RJ, et al. World Health Organization global estimates and regional comparisons of the burden of foodborne disease in 2010. PLoS Med. 2015;12(12):e1001923.
83. Truong HN, Garmyn D, Gal L, Fournier C, Sevellec Y, Jeandroz S, et al. Plants as a realized niche for Listeria monocytogenes. Microbiology. 2021;10(6):e1255.
84. Yeni F, Yavas S, Alpas H, Soyer Y. Most common foodborne pathogens and mycotoxins on fresh produce: a review of recent outbreaks. Crit Rev Food Sci Nutr. 2016;56(9):1532–44.
85. Liu Y, Wu F. Global burden of aflatoxin-induced hepatocellular carcinoma: a risk assessment. Environ Health Perspect. 2010;118(6):818–24.

Chapter 9
Shellfish Allergy and Intoxication

Angulo Romero Heidy, Pérez Herazo Juan, Amell Salas Dana, Badel Dávila Ana, Meléndez Diaz Luis, and Brito Fragoso Ana María

Introduction

The intake of food and the health status of the population are intimately related. What people consume has a direct influence on exposure to foodborne pathogens, allergens, environmental contaminants, and even the occurrence of acute events such as intoxications and allergies. All of this is interrelated with a complex network of factors, such as socioeconomic status, food accessibility, preferences, culture, and politics, among others [1].

Foodborne diseases (FBD) constitute one of the most widespread issues globally. The World Health Organization (WHO) estimates that 1 in 10 people is affected annually by consuming contaminated food, with approximately 420,000 deaths. Moreover, FBDs are a fundamental cause of decreased productivity for nations, organizations, families, and individuals [2]. FBDs can be classified into infections, intoxications, or toxin-mediated infections. Foodborne infections result from ingesting food containing live pathogenic microorganisms, such as *Salmonella*, *Shigella*, hepatitis A virus, *Trichinella spiralis*, among others. On the other hand, food intoxication occurs when toxins produced by bacteria or molds are present in the ingested food or when there are chemical substances in harmful quantities. Generally, toxins have no odor or taste and can cause illness even after the microorganisms have been eliminated, constituting a case of toxin-mediated infection [3].

A. R. Heidy (✉)
Universidad del Sinú, Cartagena, Colombia

P. H. Juan · A. S. Dana · B. D. Ana · M. D. Luis · B. F. A. María
Corporación Universitaria Rafael Núñez, Faculty of Health Sciences, School of Medicine, GINUMED Research Group, Cartagena, Bolívar, Colombia
e-mail: jperezh10@curnvirtual.edu.co; damells10@curnvirtual.edu.co; abadeld10@curnvirtual.edu.co; abritof10@curnvirtual.edu.co

M. G. Múnera Gómez et al. (eds.), *Allergies, Poisoning and Intolerance to Common Substances*, https://doi.org/10.1007/978-3-031-93658-6_9

Food consumption is also closely related to the development of food allergies, which, according to the National Institute of Allergy and Infectious Diseases and the European Academy of Allergy and Clinical Immunology, are defined as an "adverse reaction to certain foods that arises from a specific immune response, whether mediated by immunoglobulin (Ig) E, cells, or both" [4]. Worldwide, approximately 520 million people may suffer from food allergies. According to data from the World Allergy Organization, no country has reported a decrease in food allergies in the past 10 years. In Europe, more than 17 million people suffer from this type of allergy, of which approximately 3.5 million are under 25 years old, making it the leading cause of anaphylaxis in children aged 0–14 years [5].

Shellfish Allergy

Shellfish allergy is one of the most common worldwide and is considered one of the main causes of food-induced anaphylaxis. Adults have a higher prevalence of shellfish allergy than the pediatric population; however, this type of allergy often appears in late childhood or adolescence and is believed to persist for life in up to 90% of patients. Shellfish allergies tend to present as anaphylaxis or potentially life-threatening episodes, with shrimp and crab being the main causes of anaphylaxis in both children and adults. Edible shellfish are divided into three phyla: arthropods, mollusks, and fish. Edible mollusks can be divided into three classes: gastropods, bivalves, and cephalopods. Edible arthropods belong to the subphylum Crustacea, specifically the order Decapoda, which includes prawns, shrimp, crabs, and lobsters. Among fish, allergies have a higher prevalence in bony fish, while cartilaginous fish tend to have a lower prevalence [6, 7].

Adverse reactions to shellfish can be classified into three categories based on their mechanism: IgE-mediated and non-IgE-mediated immune reactions, toxic reactions (such as those caused by marine biotoxins), and food intolerance. Adverse reactions due to toxins or food intolerance can have clinical characteristics similar to shellfish allergy. Symptoms due to allergies after ingestion can present within minutes and include nausea, vomiting, hives, asthma exacerbation, and anaphylaxis. Respiratory reactions, along with oral allergy syndrome, are frequently reported in shellfish allergy. Sensitization and subsequent reactions occur more frequently after ingestion; however, they can also occur due to skin contact or inhalation of aerosolized proteins generated during cooking or processing in factories and domestic environments [8] (Fig. 9.1).

The main shellfish allergens involved in the development of these allergies are high-molecular-weight, thermostable proteins that are not inactivated by cooking. This process can increase the allergenicity of shellfish through mechanisms such as protein denaturation, exposure to new epitopes, aggregation, and chemical modification [9]. Among the allergens are tropomyosin, arginine kinase, myosin light chain, sarcoplasmic calcium-binding protein, hemocyanin, and troponin C [8].

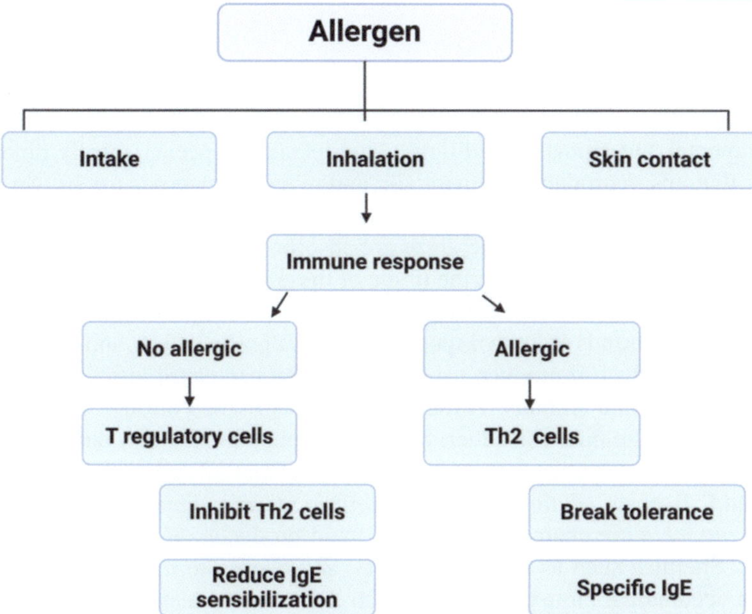

Fig. 9.1 Allergens can enter the body through various routes, such as ingestion, inhalation, or skin contact, triggering an immune response. In non-allergic individuals, regulatory T cells inhibit the Th2 response, preventing IgE sensitization. In contrast, allergic individuals have antigen-specific Th2 cells that lead to a breakdown of immune tolerance. This results in the production of specific IgE, which is responsible for allergic reactions. Thus, the immune system responds differently depending on the individual's allergic predisposition

As with any IgE-mediated immune reaction, the process begins with the absorption of antigens through the intestinal epithelium (ingestion), pulmonary mucosa (inhalation), or skin (contact). In a non-allergic individual, after allergen absorption, regulatory T cells are generated through tolerance mechanisms involving dendritic cells and macrophages. These T cells inhibit the Th2 response and prevent the development of IgE sensitization. However, in allergic (atopic) patients, this process fails because antigen-presenting cells induce a Th2 response, with IL-4 playing a key role in inducing the formation of Th2 cells specific to the presented antigen. This leads to the breakdown of tolerance and the production of antigen-specific IgE, which binds to IgE surface receptors on mast cells/basophils, as shown in Fig. 9.1 [10].

Re-exposure to the antigen and the binding and cross-linking of allergen-specific IgE on mast cells and basophils lead to degranulation, the release of preformed granules containing tryptase and histamine, and the development of new mediators such as prostaglandins and leukotrienes. These effects involve vasodilation, mucus secretion, smooth muscle contraction, and chemotaxis of other inflammatory cells, which sustain and amplify the inflammatory process, causing the clinical manifestations characteristic of allergic reactions [11].

Shellfish Intoxication

Marine biotoxins are described as natural chemical substances primarily produced by phytoplankton. The global presence of biotoxins is correlated with favorable environmental and climatic conditions. Phytoplankton species, mostly dinoflagellates or diatoms, reproduce exponentially and release dangerous toxins. An important cause of adverse reactions to seafood is the presence of numerous toxins in fish, crustaceans, and mollusks. Toxic algae are absorbed by filter feeders such as mussels and oysters, accumulated in the tissue of these invertebrates, and consumed by fish that absorb some of these toxins [12].

There are thousands of known species of microalgae in nature, and it is estimated that approximately 100 produce natural toxins that can cause intoxication or even death in humans and animals. These toxins are distributed through the food chain until they reach the final consumer: humans. Human intoxication outbreaks due to marine biotoxins can have a wide range of symptoms related to the specific toxic compound. Species of the genera *Alexandria*, *Gymnodinium*, *Dinophysis*, and *Pseudo-nitzschia* are characterized as the main producers of marine biotoxins for humans. Shellfish such as mussels, oysters, and clams are filter-feeding mollusks that can accumulate biotoxins according to their natural habits in the food chain. Consumer exposure to these toxins depends on the number of shellfish consumed and the amount of toxin present in the shellfish. Most of these toxins have a phytoplanktonic origin and bioaccumulate primarily in the tissues of shellfish after filtering toxic microalgae. Many marine organisms, in addition to bivalve mollusks, can act as vectors for toxins, such as echinoderms, tunicates, marine gastropods, or crustaceans [13] (Table 9.1).

Table 9.1 A summary of the various types of reactions to shellfish consumption, their causes, mechanisms of action, and associated symptoms

Type of reaction	Cause	Mechanism of action	Symptoms
Shellfish allergy	IgE-mediated allergens	Immune response involving IgE, Th2 cells, and B cells	Nausea, vomiting, hives, asthma exacerbation, anaphylaxis
Amnesic shellfish poisoning	Domoic acid	Binds to glutamate receptors, causing neurotoxicity	Nausea, vomiting, diarrhea, confusion, memory loss, seizures
Diarrhetic shellfish poisoning	Okadaic acid, dinophysistoxins	Inhibition of serine/threonine phosphoprotein phosphatases	Nausea, vomiting, diarrhea
Neurotoxic shellfish poisoning	Brevetoxins	Acts on voltage-gated sodium channels	Nausea, vomiting, diarrhea, numbness, tingling, coordination problems
Paralytic shellfish poisoning	Saxitoxins	Blocks voltage-gated sodium channels	Numbness, tingling, headache, dizziness, paralysis, respiratory arrest

Toxicokinetics

Consumption of shellfish can lead to various types of intoxications. Five main groups of syndromes are described [14].

Amnesic Shellfish Poisoning

Amnesic shellfish poisoning is caused by a potent neurotoxin called domoic acid (DA), also known as amnesic shellfish toxin. The genus of marine diatoms *Pseudo-nitzschia* is widely distributed internationally and comprises 48 popular species; at least 23 of them are known to be potential producers of DA [15]. DA is structurally similar to glutamic acid and acts as an agonist. It is a potent neuroexcitant that binds strongly to glutamate receptors in the brain tissue, particularly in the hippocampus, significantly interfering with synapses, causing calcium channel opening, and leading to neuronal necrosis due to calcium overload [16].

Diarrhetic Shellfish Poisoning

Diarrhetic shellfish poisoning is produced by marine dinoflagellates belonging to the genera *Dinophysis* and *Prorocentrum*. Diarrhetic shellfish toxins include okadaic acid (OA) and dinophysistoxins (DTX) and their derivatives. These lipophilic molecules are among the most frequently reported marine toxins in Europe, Asia, and South America [17]. The mechanism of action involved in this type of intoxication is the inhibition of serine/threonine phosphoprotein phosphatases. This group of toxins is a significant cause of gastrointestinal dysfunction, clinically manifesting as nausea, vomiting, and diarrhea [18].

Neurotoxic Shellfish Poisoning

Neurotoxic shellfish poisoning results from ingesting shellfish contaminated with brevetoxins (BTX), which are chemically characterized by their ladder-like cyclic ether structures with trans/syn-fused ether rings. Their primary mechanism of action is on voltage-gated sodium channels. These toxins are secreted by algal blooms and accumulate in the bodies of shellfish [19].

Paralytic Shellfish Poisoning

Paralytic shellfish poisoning is caused by saxitoxins, which are alkaloids produced by dinoflagellates of the genera *Alexandrium*, *Gymnodinium*, or *Pyrodinium*, or by certain cyanobacteria. The toxins typically accumulate in mussels, crabs that eat mussels, or certain fish. Their neurotoxic mechanism blocks sodium channels in the nervous system, acting extremely quickly (10–15 min after consuming contaminated shellfish) [20]. The neurotoxic action of paralytic shellfish toxins results from blocking voltage-gated sodium channels, leading to a progressive loss of neuromuscular functions. Symptoms vary from mild neurological and gastrointestinal effects to death from respiratory arrest [21].

Azaspiracid Poisoning (AZP)

Azaspiracids are produced by dinoflagellates of the genera *Azadinium* and *Amphidoma*, causing intoxications after consuming contaminated seafood, especially mussels [22]. Azaspiracids have unusual dynamics, resulting in unpredictable and temporary intoxication patterns. They accumulate in bivalve mollusks that feed on toxic microalgae. AZP may be widespread but often goes unreported due to similarities with diarrheic shellfish poisoning and bacterial enterotoxin intoxication [23].

Due to the broad spectrum of mechanisms causing shellfish allergy and intoxication, clinical manifestations in patients can vary. A comprehensive evaluation should consider factors such as the onset and progression of symptoms, as shown in Table 9.1.

Food intake is a human biological necessity that generates the demand for food products, whether fresh or processed. Fishing, and especially aquaculture production, has significantly contributed to the global supply of fish, crustaceans, mollusks, and other aquatic organisms. Since 2000, this trend has been increasing, with the global production of fish and seafood estimated to have reached approximately 179 million tons in 2018, with a total value of 401 billion dollars, and aquaculture accounting for 46% of the total production [24].

Collective and individual preferences for the consumption of seafood products have contributed to a significant increase in reports of intoxications caused by their consumption. This can be influenced by the lack of preservation in food safety, a complex process that starts at aquaculture exploitation and ends with the consumer. The consumer also has the responsibility to take the necessary hygiene measures to ensure this safety. Regarding allergic reactions, they have an important genetic component that must be considered.

Glossary

Glossary of Acronyms

DA Domoic acid
DTX Dinophysistoxins
FBD Foodborne diseases
IgE Immunoglobulin E
IL-4 Interleukin 4
OA Okadaic acid
PSP Paralytic shellfish poisoning
Th2 T-helper 2 (cells)
WHO World Health Organization
AZP Azaspiracid poisoning

Glossary of Terms

Adverse Reaction An unwanted or harmful reaction experienced following the administration of a substance or exposure to a factor.
Anaphylaxis A severe, potentially life-threatening allergic reaction that can occur rapidly.
Aquaculture The breeding, rearing, and harvesting of fish, shellfish, algae, and other organisms in all types of water environments.
Biotoxin A toxic substance produced by a living organism, often found in marine environments.
Dinoflagellate A type of plankton that is often associated with harmful algal blooms and the production of toxins.
Echinoderms A phylum of marine animals including starfish and sea urchins that can act as vectors for toxins.
Foodborne Disease (FBD) An illness caused by consuming contaminated food.
Immunoglobulin E (IgE) A class of antibodies produced by the immune system in response to allergens.
Paralytic Shellfish Poisoning (PSP) A condition caused by consuming shellfish contaminated with saxitoxins, which block sodium channels.
Phytoplankton Microscopic marine algae that form the basis of the aquatic food web and can produce biotoxins.

References

1. Majowicz SE, Meyer SB, Kirkpatrick SI, Graham JL, Shaikh A, Elliott SJ, et al. Food, health, and complexity: towards a conceptual understanding to guide collaborative public health action. BMC Public Health [Internet]. 2016 Jun 8 [cited 2022 Dec 1];16(1). Available from: https://pmc.ncbi.nlm.nih.gov/articles/PMC4898364/.
2. Dueñas Moreira O, Puig Peña Y, Romero Placeres M, Gámez Sánchez D, Puñales Sosa OV, Leyva Castillo V. Perfil del riesgo de brotes alimentarios por intoxicación estafilocócica en Cuba [Internet]. 2021. Available from: https://orcid.org/0000-0002-4019-3009.
3. OPS/OMS | Enfermedades transmitidas por alimentos (ETA) [Internet]. [cited 2022 Dec 4]. Available from: https://www3.paho.org/hq/index.php?option=com_content&view=article&id=10836:2015-enfermedades-transmitidas-por-alimentos-eta&Itemid=0&lang=es#gsc.tab=0.
4. Reyes-Pavón D, Jiménez M, Salinas E, Reyes-Pavón D, Jiménez M, Salinas E. Fisiopatología de la alergia alimentaria. Rev Alerg Mex [Internet]. 2020 [cited 2022 Dec 4];67(1):34–53. Available from: http://www.scielo.org.mx/scielo.php?script=sci_arttext&pid=S2448-91902020000100034&lng=es&nrm=iso&tlng=es.
5. Incidencia de la alergia alimentaria – Fundación FSA [Internet]. [cited 2022 Dec 4]. Available from: https://funsapa.org/alergia-alimentaria/incidencia/
6. Wong L, Tham EH, Lee BW. An update on shellfish allergy. Vol. 19, Curr Opin Allergy Clin Immunol. Lippincott Williams and Wilkins; 2019. p. 236–242.
7. Ruethers T, Taki AC, Johnston EB, Nugraha R, Le TTK, Kalic T, et al. Seafood allergy: a comprehensive review of fish and shellfish allergens. Mol Immunol. 2018;100:28–57.
8. Davis CM, Gupta RS, Aktas ON, Diaz V, Kamath SD, Lopata AL. Clinical management of seafood allergy. J Allergy Clin Immunol Pract. 2020;8(1):37–44.
9. Prester L. Seafood allergy, toxicity, and intolerance: a review. J Am Coll Nutr [Internet]. 2016 [cited 2022 Dec 1];35(3):271–83. Available from: https://pubmed.ncbi.nlm.nih.gov/26252073/.
10. Buyuktiryaki B, Masini M, Mori F, Barni S, Liccioli G, Sarti L, et al. Ige-mediated fish allergy in children. Medicina (Lithuania) MDPI AG. 2021;57:1–22.
11. Pali-Schöll I, Untersmayr E, Klems M, Jensen-Jarolim E. The effect of digestion and digestibility on allergenicity of food. Nutrients [Internet]. 2018 [cited 2022 Dec 1];10(9). Available from: https://pmc.ncbi.nlm.nih.gov/articles/PMC6164088/
12. Nicolas J, Hoogenboom RLAP, Hendriksen PJM, Bodero M, Bovee TFH, Rietjens IMCM, et al. Marine biotoxins and associated outbreaks following seafood consumption: prevention and surveillance in the 21st century. Global Food Secur Elsevier B.V. 2017;15:11–21.
13. Farabegoli F, Blanco L, Rodríguez LP, Manuel Vieites J, García Cabado A. Phycotoxins in marine shellfish: origin, occurrence and effects on humans. Marine Drugs MDPI AG. 2018;16
14. Costa PR, Marques A, Diogène J. Marine biotoxins and seafood poisoning. Toxins (Basel) [Internet]. 2019 [cited 2022 Jul 26];11(10). Available from: https://pubmed.ncbi.nlm.nih.gov/31554162/.
15. Montoya NG, Carignan MO, Mattera MB. Toxinas Algales en el Mar Argentino: nuevos hallazgos, nuevos desafíos. Acta toxicol argent [Internet]. 2020 [cited 2022 Dec 1];21–30. Available from: http://www.scielo.org.ar/scielo.php?script=sci_arttext&pid=S1851-37432020000300021.
16. Alvarez-Falconí PP. Ácido domoico e intoxicación amnésica por moluscos en salud pública. Rev Peru Med Exp Salud Publica [Internet]. 2009 [cited 2022 Dec 1];26(4):505–16. Available from: http://www.scielo.org.pe/scielo.php?script=sci_arttext&pid=S1726-46342009000400013&lng=es&nrm=iso&tlng=es.
17. Louzao MC, Vilariño N, Vale C, Costas C, Cao A, Raposo-garcia S, et al. Current trends and new challenges in marine phycotoxins. Mar Drugs [Internet]. 2022 [cited 2022 Dec 1];20(3). Available from: https://pubmed.ncbi.nlm.nih.gov/35323497/.

18. Reguera B, Riobó P, Rodríguez F, Díaz PA, Pizarro G, Paz B, et al. Dinophysis toxins: causative organisms, distribution and fate in Shellfish. Mar Drugs [Internet]. 2014 [cited 2022 Dec 1];12(1):394. Available from: https://pmc.ncbi.nlm.nih.gov/articles/PMC3917280/.
19. Kalaitzis JA, Chau R, Kohli GS, Murray SA, Neilan BA. Biosynthesis of toxic naturally-occurring seafood contaminants. Toxicon. 2010;56(2):244–58.
20. Hess P. Poisoning caused by marine biotoxins. Bundesgesundheitsblatt Gesundheitsforschung Gesundheitsschutz [Internet]. 2017 [cited 2022 Dec 1];60(7):757–60. Available from: https://link.springer.com/article/10.1007/s00103-017-2562-5.
21. Arnich N, Thébault A. Dose-response modelling of paralytic shellfish poisoning (PSP) in humans. Toxins (Basel) [Internet]. 2018 [cited 2022 Dec 1];10(4). Available from: https://pmc.ncbi.nlm.nih.gov/articles/PMC5923307/.
22. Boente-Juncal A, Raposo-García S, Louzao MC, Vale C, Botana LM. Targeting chloride ion channels: new insights into the mechanism of action of the marine toxin Azaspiracid. Chem Res Toxicol [Internet]. 2021 Mar 15 [cited 2022 Dec 1];34(3):865–79. Available from: https://pubmed.ncbi.nlm.nih.gov/33512997/.
23. Furey A, O'Doherty S, O'Callaghan K, Lehane M, James KJ. Azaspiracid poisoning (AZP) toxins in shellfish: toxicological and health considerations. Toxicon. 2010;56(2):173–90.
24. Basilio O, Zaragoza DR, Tanahara S, Lugo-Ibarra KC, Miroslava VA. Study of consumer perceptions and preferences: consumption case study of fish and shellfish in Mexicali, Baja California, Mexico. [cited 2022 Dec 4]; Available from: https://www.researchgate.net/publication/356645935.

Chapter 10
Meat Poisoning and Allergy

Marlon Gustavo Múnera Gómez, Sathya Arenas, Valeria Gratz, and Juana Bustillo Arias

Introduction

Food poisoning is a public health issue of global scope that affects millions of people around the world each year. Among the various sources of food contamination, the consumption of raw or undercooked meat poses a significant health risk due to its potential to harbor a variety of dangerous pathogens [1]. From bacteria to parasites, these microorganisms can cause serious illnesses ranging from gastroenteritis to more severe syndromes like hemolytic uremic syndrome (HUS) [2].

In this chapter, we will explain in detail the main pathogens associated with food poisoning from beef, chicken, pork, fish, and processed meats, as well as the management and treatment strategies for each type of poisoning. From the well-known *Escherichia coli* O157 to the feared *Salmonella*, we will analyze the prevalence, clinical symptoms, and potential complications associated with each of these pathogenic agents.

M. G. Múnera Gómez (✉)
Corporación Universitaria Rafael Núñez, GINUMED Group, Cartagena, Bolívar, Colombia
e-mail: vgrattzl10@curnvirtual.edu.co

S. Arenas
Universidad del Sinú, Faculty of Health, Cartagena, Colombia

V. Gratz
Corporación Universitaria Rafael Núñez, Faculty of Health, Cartagena, Bolívar, Colombia
e-mail: vgrattzl10@curnvirtual.edu.co

J. B. Arias
Neuroinmune, Research Department, Cartagena, Colombia

M. G. Múnera Gómez et al. (eds.), *Allergies, Poisoning and Intolerance to Common Substances*, https://doi.org/10.1007/978-3-031-93658-6_10

Most Common Pathogens in Meat Poisoning

There is significant etiological variety in meat poisoning (beef, chicken, fish, pork, ground meat, and processed meats), which necessitates targeted management based on the causative agent [3]. This etiological diversity arises from several factors, including:

- Different production and processing practices: Each type of meat may be subject to different production, processing, and distribution practices, influencing the types of pathogens that can contaminate it. For instance, fish can be exposed to waterborne pathogens like *Vibrio* spp., while red meats may be more exposed to soil or environmentally transmitted pathogens [3, 4].
- Contamination at various stages: Meat can become contaminated with pathogens at various stages of the food chain, from farm to table. This can include contamination during slaughter, processing, transportation, storage, and food preparation [3].
- Differences in natural microbiota: Each type of meat may have a unique natural microbiota that influences its susceptibility to pathogen contamination. For example, beef can harbor *E. coli* in the cattle's gastrointestinal tract, while fish may be exposed to waterborne pathogens in its natural environment [3, 5].

  – Variability in cooking practices: The way different types of meat are prepared and cooked can vary, which in turn can influence the effectiveness of eliminating or reducing pathogen load. For example, ground meat may have a greater surface area exposed to potential pathogens, while processed meats may contain additional ingredients that could introduce contamination [3].
  – Differences in susceptibility to certain pathogens: Some types of meat may be more susceptible than others to certain pathogens due to their intrinsic characteristics, such as water content, pH, and the presence of nutrients that promote bacterial growth [3].

According to the above, there are several microorganisms that can contaminate and cause food poisoning in different types of meat, such as *Salmonella*, *Listeria*, *Campylobacter*, and *Escherichia coli*, along with others that are more specific, such as *Vibrio* in fish and *Yersinia* in pork. (Table 10.1).

Table 10.1 Main pathogens derived from meat poisoning

Main pathogens associated with meat poisoning	
Type of meat	Type of meat
Beef	*Escherichia coli* (e.g., O157), *Salmonella*
Chicken	*Campylobacter*, *Salmonella*
Pork	*Yersinia enterocolitica*, *Salmonella*
Fish	*Vibrio* spp., *Listeria monocytogenes*
Ground meat	*Escherichia coli*, *Salmonella*
Processed meat	*Listeria monocytogenes*, *Salmonella*

Escherichia coli *O157*

It is a pathogenic strain of *E. coli* characterized by the production of toxins, including Shiga toxin, and its ability to cause severe illnesses in humans, such as bloody diarrhea and hemolytic uremic syndrome (HUS) [6]. This strain is identified by its O157 serotype, which is crucial for accurate diagnosis. These distinctive microbiological characteristics make *E. coli* O157 a significant concern in terms of public health and food safety.

E. coli O157 can contaminate various types of meat, but beef, particularly ground beef, is noted as a common source of this contamination. This is due to the presence of *E. coli* O157 in the intestinal tract of cattle, which can contaminate meat during slaughter and processing stages [7]. Additionally, there is a risk of contamination during the meat processing and packaging, increasing the likelihood of this bacterium being present in meat products [8].

The management of *E. coli* O157 poisoning varies depending on the severity of the symptoms. In mild cases, rehydration and symptom control may be recommended, whereas in more severe situations, such as the development of hemolytic uremic syndrome (HUS), hospitalization may be necessary, which could include blood transfusions and renal dialysis [9].

It is crucial to emphasize that prevention is key to avoiding *E. coli* O157 poisoning. It is recommended to cook meat to a safe temperature to eliminate the bacteria, maintain good personal and kitchen utensil hygiene, and avoid consuming raw or undercooked meat. Additionally, it is essential to follow proper hygiene and food safety practices at all stages of food production, processing, and handling to reduce the risk of *E. coli* O157 contamination [10, 11].

Salmonella

Salmonella is a genus of Gram-negative, facultatively anaerobic, motile bacteria due to their peritrichous flagella, and they are non-spore-forming. The cells are straight or slightly curved bacilli, measuring 2–5 micrometers in length and 0.5–1.5 micrometers in width. This bacterium can survive in harsh environments, such as dry and low-humidity foods, and it can withstand the acidity of the human stomach. Additionally, *Salmonella* can form biofilms, allowing it to adhere to surfaces and protect itself from disinfectants and antibiotics [12].

Salmonella is most frequently found in poultry, such as chickens and turkeys, as well as in products derived from these birds, such as eggs. Pork meat has also been noted to be at risk of *Salmonella* contamination. It is important to highlight that consuming raw or undercooked meat increases the risk of contracting *Salmonella* [13, 14].

The management of meat poisoning caused by *Salmonella* primarily involves supportive measures and, in severe cases, antibiotic treatment. In most instances, *Salmonella* infection is self-limiting and does not require specific treatment.

However, for patients with severe symptoms or those with compromised immune systems, antibiotics may be considered to control the infection [15].

The treatment of *Salmonella* poisoning includes supportive measures such as oral or intravenous rehydration to prevent dehydration caused by diarrhea. Additionally, medications can be administered to control symptoms such as fever and diarrhea [12].

It is crucial for patients to avoid self-medicating with antibiotics, as improper use can contribute to the development of bacterial resistance. Therefore, antibiotic treatment should be supervised according to the progression of symptoms and, ideally, guided by culture results (in this case, stool cultures) [16].

To prevent *Salmonella* poisoning from meat, it is crucial to cook animal-based foods to safe temperatures to eliminate the bacteria. Additionally, proper food hygiene practices should be followed, such as regularly washing hands and kitchen utensils and avoiding cross-contamination between raw and cooked foods [17].

Listeria Monocytogenes

Listeria monocytogenes is a facultative, non-spore-forming, anaerobic bacterium with flagella that confer motility. It stains positive in Gram staining and has a bacillary shape, being oxidase-negative and catalase-positive. This bacterium can form biofilms and has been identified in various environments, such as soil, water, vegetation, drains, and animal and human feces [12].

Listeria monocytogenes has been detected in a variety of meat products, including beef cuts, chicken, and processed meats like mortadella, salami, and prosciutto [18].

The management of *Listeria monocytogenes* poisoning depends on the severity of symptoms and the patient's condition. In mild cases, symptoms may resolve without specific treatment. However, in patients with severe symptoms or those in high-risk groups—such as pregnant women, newborns, the elderly, or immunocompromised individuals—antibiotic administration is recommended. The antibiotics of choice are typically ampicillin or penicillin G, and in cases of allergy to these, trimethoprim-sulfamethoxazole can be considered as an alternative. It is essential to seek medical attention to assess the need for treatment and closely monitor the patient's progress, especially in high-risk groups, to prevent severe complications associated with *Listeria monocytogenes* infection [19].

Campylobacter

The genus *Campylobacter* is characterized as a group of Gram-negative bacteria with a short, curved morphology. They are oxidase-positive and microaerophilic. These bacteria are part of the commensal microbiota of the gastrointestinal tract of humans, domestic animals, and wildlife, particularly avian species. Additionally, *Campylobacter* utilizes tricarboxylic acid cycle intermediates and amino acids as energy substrates, unlike other bacteria that undergo carbohydrate fermentation or oxidation [20, 21, 22].

Poultry meat, especially chicken, is the primary source of *Campylobacter* infection in humans, with an estimated 50–80% of infection cases attributed to the consumption of contaminated chicken meat. Furthermore, it has been documented that beef, pork, and raw milk can also serve as sources of *Campylobacter* infection [22].

The therapeutic approach for a patient with *Vibrio* poisoning depends on the severity of symptoms and the extent of the infection. In mild cases, treatment may involve supportive measures such as adequate hydration and rest. In more severe cases, treatment with specific antibiotics may be necessary to combat the infection [4].

Some of the antibiotics commonly used to treat *Vibrio* infections include ciprofloxacin, doxycycline, azithromycin, and third-generation cephalosporins. It is important to note that certain types of *Vibrio* can be resistant to specific antibiotics, making culture-guided therapy often necessary to determine the most effective treatment. Additionally, in cases of severe or systemic infection, hospitalization with intensive medical monitoring and support may be required [23].

In general, prevention is the best strategy to avoid *Vibrio* poisoning. It is recommended to cook food properly, especially seafood, and to avoid the consumption of raw or undercooked shellfish. Maintaining good personal and food hygiene is also important, as well as avoiding contact with contaminated seawater or exposing open wounds while swimming in the sea.

Introduction to Meat Allergy

Meat allergy, although historically considered rare, has gained significant attention in recent decades. There are several types of meat allergies, including those mediated by IgE and others with less conventional mechanisms. The most studied types include primary beef allergy, pork-cat syndrome, and alpha-gal syndrome (AGS).

Types and Mechanisms of Meat Allergies

1. Primary Beef Allergy: Commonly observed in atopic children, this form of allergy is associated with sensitization to proteins such as bovine serum albumin (Bos d 6). Symptoms are usually immediate and range from urticaria to anaphylaxis [24].
2. Pork-Cat Syndrome: This involves sensitization to cat serum albumin (Fel d 2), which can lead to reactions upon consuming pork products due to cross-reactivity with pork serum albumin (Sus s 1). This highlights the importance of prior respiratory sensitization [25].

3. Alpha-Gal Syndrome (AGS): First identified in 2009, AGS is an IgE-mediated allergy to the oligosaccharide galactose-alpha-1,3-galactose (alpha-gal), found in non-primate mammalian tissues. Sensitization is typically related to tick bites, particularly from *Amblyomma americanum* (lone star tick). This allergy is notable for delayed reactions, usually appearing 3–6 h after consuming mammalian meat [26].

Immunological Mechanisms and Sensitization

- Sensitization to Alpha-Gal: Sensitization occurs after tick bites introduce saliva containing alpha-gal epitopes, which trigger a Th2-type immune response. This response stimulates the production of alpha-gal-specific IgE, leading to allergic reactions upon the consumption of mammalian meat [27].
- Immunological Features: AGS reactions involve the activation of mast cells and basophils, releasing allergic mediators such as histamine. The delayed onset of symptoms may be explained by the digestion and metabolism of alpha-gal-containing glycolipids and glycoproteins.

Epidemiology and Regional Distribution

AGS is more prevalent in regions where the ticks that trigger sensitization are common, such as the southeastern United States. Cases have also been reported in Europe, Australia, and other areas where different tick species can induce sensitization [28].

Diagnosis and Management

Diagnosis of AGS involves identifying specific IgE to alpha-gal and a compatible clinical history. Management includes avoiding mammalian-derived products and using antihistamines and mast cell stabilizers to control symptoms [29].

Conclusion

Meat poisoning represents a significant public health challenge due to the variety of pathogens that can contaminate these foods. From bacteria such as *Escherichia coli* O157:H7, *Salmonella*, *Listeria monocytogenes*, and *Campylobacter* to the *Vibrio* genus mainly associated with seafood, each poses specific risks to human health. These microorganisms can contaminate meat at various stages of the food chain, from production and processing to preparation and final consumption.

The severity of poisoning varies depending on the pathogen and the susceptibility of the affected individual, with symptoms ranging from mild gastroenteritis to serious illnesses such as hemolytic uremic syndrome or neonatal complications. Treatment also varies, from supportive measures and symptom management to the administration of antibiotics in severe cases.

Prevention plays a crucial role in reducing the risk of meat poisoning. Measures emphasized include properly cooking food, maintaining good personal hygiene and clean kitchen utensils, avoiding the consumption of raw or undercooked meat, and following proper food hygiene and safety practices at all stages of production and handling.

In summary, meat poisoning is a complex issue that requires a comprehensive approach encompassing everything from production to consumption, with a strong emphasis on prevention through proper food handling and preparation practices.

Glossary

Glossary of Acronyms

BAT Basophil Activation Test
CBD Cannabidiol
CB1 Cannabinoid Receptor 1
CB2 Cannabinoid Receptor 2
GINUMED Group of Medicine Investigation
GIFTCA Pharmaceutical Cosmetic and Food Technology Research Group
IUIS International Union of Immunological Societies
LTP Lipid Transfer Protein
OEEP2 Oxygen-Evolving Enhancer Protein 2
PPARγ Peroxisome Proliferator-Activated Receptor Gamma
PR10 Pathogenesis-Related Protein 10
pMAT Mast Cell Activation Test
Pru p 3 Lipid Transfer Protein from Peach
rCan s 3 Recombinant Can s 3
RuBisCO Ribulose-1,5-bisphosphate carboxylase/oxygenase
SPT Skin Prick Test
THC Tetrahydrocannabinol
TRPV1 Transient Receptor Potential Vanilloid 1
UGT UDP-Glucuronosyltransferase
WHO World Health Organization

Glossary of Terms

Food Allergy An adverse immune response to proteins in meat, mediated by IgE or non-IgE mechanisms.

Basophil Activation Test (BAT) A test that measures basophil activation to diagnose food allergies.

Cross-Reactivity A phenomenon where structurally similar proteins from different species trigger an immune response.

Lipid Transfer Protein (LTP) Proteins resistant to digestion that act as common allergens in foods, including some meats.

Mast Cell Activation Test (pMAT) An in vitro test that measures mast cell activation in response to allergens.

Histamine A substance released by mast cells during an allergic reaction, responsible for symptoms like itching and inflammation.

Immunoglobulin E (IgE) An antibody involved in immune-mediated allergic reactions.

Anisakis simplex A parasite that can cause allergic reactions when consuming contaminated fish or meat.

Skin Prick Test (SPT) A diagnostic method to identify allergies by exposing the skin to allergenic extracts.

Recombinant Proteins (rCan s 3) Synthetic proteins used in diagnostic tests to detect sensitization to specific allergens.

References

1. Dlamini BS, Montso PK, Kumar A, Ateba CN. Distribution of virulence factors, determinants of antibiotic resistance and molecular fingerprinting of Salmonella species isolated from cattle and beef samples: suggestive evidence of animal-to-meat contamination. Environ Sci Pollut Res. 2018;25(32):32694–708.
2. Amani MA, Sarkodie SA. Mitigating spread of contamination in meat supply chain management using deep learning. Sci Rep. 2022;12(1):5037.
3. Murray A. Meat cultures: Lab-grown meat and the politics of contamination. BioSocieties. 2018;13(2):513–34.
4. El-Zamkan MA, Ahmed AS, Abdelhafeez HH, Mohamed HMA. Molecular characterization of Vibrio species isolated from dairy and water samples. Sci Rep. 2023;13(1)
5. Ayoade F, Oguzie J, Eromon P, Omotosho OE, Ogunbiyi T, Olumade T, et al. Molecular surveillance of shiga toxigenic Escherichia coli in selected beef abattoirs in Osun State Nigeria. Sci Rep. 2021;11(1):13966.
6. Zhang D, Coronel-Aguilera CP, Romero PL, Perry L, Minocha U, Rosenfield C, et al. The use of a novel NanoLuc-based reporter phage for the detection of Escherichia coli O157:H7. Sci Rep. 2016;6
7. Alhadlaq MA, Mujallad MI, Alajel SMI. Detection of Escherichia coli O157:H7 in imported meat products from Saudi Arabian ports in 2017. Sci Rep. 2023;13(1)
8. Guragain M, Schmidt JW, Kalchayanand N, Dickey AM, Bosilevac JM. Characterization of Escherichia coli harboring colibactin genes (clb) isolated from beef production and processing systems. Sci Rep. 2022;12(1):5305.

9. Darphorn TS, Bel K, Koenders-van Sint Anneland BB, Brul S, Ter Kuile BH. Antibiotic resistance plasmid composition and architecture in Escherichia coli isolates from meat. Sci Rep. 2021;11(1):2136.
10. Innes GK, Patton AN, Nachman KE, Casey JA, Stapleton GS, Abraham AG, et al. Distance and destination of retail meat alter multidrug resistant contamination in the United States food system. Sci Rep. 2023;13(1)
11. Nüesch-Inderbinen M, Treier A, Stevens MJA, Stephan R. Whole genome sequence-based characterisation of Shiga toxin-producing Escherichia coli isolated from game meat originating from several European countries. Sci Rep. 2023;13(1):3247.
12. Obaidat MM. Prevalence and antimicrobial resistance of Listeria monocytogenes, Salmonella enterica and Escherichia coli O157:H7 in imported beef cattle in Jordan. Comp Immunol Microbiol Infect Dis. 2020;70
13. Simon S, Lamparter MC, Pietsch M, Borowiak M, Fruth A, Rabsch W, et al. Zoonoses in food-chain animals with respect to human disease and public health relevance. In: Zoonoses: infections affecting humans and animals. Springer International Publishing; 2023. p. 1–33.
14. Kotb E, El-Nogoumy BA, Alqahtani HA, Ahmed AA, Al-shwyeh HA, Algarudi SM, et al. A putative cytotoxic serine protease from Salmonella typhimurium UcB5 recovered from undercooked burger. Sci Rep. 2023;13(1):3926.
15. Fatima A, Saleem M, Nawaz S, Khalid L, Riaz S, Sajid I. Prevalence and antibiotics resistance status of Salmonella in raw meat consumed in various areas of Lahore, Pakistan. Sci Rep. 2023;13(1):22205.
16. Ohta N, Norman KN, Norby B, Lawhon SD, Vinasco J, Den Bakker H, et al. Population dynamics of enteric Salmonella in response to antimicrobial use in beef feedlot cattle. Sci Rep. 2017;7(1):14310.
17. Yan S, Jiang Z, Zhang W, Liu Z, Dong X, Li D, et al. Genomes-based MLST, cgMLST, wgMLST and SNP analysis of salmonella Typhimurium from animals and humans. Comp Immunol Microbiol Infect Dis. 2023:96.
18. dos Santos JS, Biduski B, dos Santos LR. Listeria monocytogenes: health risk and a challenge for food processing establishments. Vol. 203, Arch Microbiol. Springer Science and Business Media Deutschland GmbH; 2021. p. 5907–5919.
19. Ravindhiran R, Sivarajan K, Sekar JN, Murugesan R, Dhandapani K. Listeria monocytogenes an emerging pathogen: a comprehensive overview on Listeriosis, virulence determinants, detection, and anti-Listerial interventions, vol. 86. Microb Ecol. Springer; 2023. p. 2231–51.
20. Rodrigues CS, Armendaris PM, de Sá CVGC, Haddad JPA, de Melo CB. Prevalence of Campylobacter spp. in chicken Carcasses in slaughterhouses from South of Brazil. Curr Microbiol. 2021;78(6):2242–50.
21. Mor-Mur M, Yuste J. Emerging bacterial pathogens in meat and poultry: an overview, vol. 3. Food Bioprocess Technol; 2010. p. 24–35.
22. Lekshmi M, Kumar SH, Nayak BB, Varela MF. Antimicrobial resistance in food-borne Campylobacter spp. In: Handbook on antimicrobial resistance. Singapore: Springer Nature; 2023. p. 1–19.
23. You HJ, Lee JH, Oh M, Hong SY, Kim D, Noh J, et al. Tackling Vibrio parahaemolyticus in ready-to-eat raw fish flesh slices using lytic phage VPT02 isolated from market oyster. Food Res Int. 2021;150
24. Wilson JM, Platts-Mills TAE. Meat allergy and allergens. Mol Immunol. 2018;100:107–12. https://doi.org/10.1016/j.molimm.2018.03.018. Epub 2018 Apr 21. PMID: 29685461; PMCID: PMC6716155
25. Perusko M, Grundström J, Eldh M, Hamsten C, Apostolovic D, van Hage M. The a-Gal epitope – the cause of a global allergic disease. Front Immunol. 2024;15:1335911. https://doi.org/10.3389/fimmu.2024.1335911.
26. Wilson JM, Platts-Mills TAE. Red meat allergy in children and adults. Curr Opin Allergy Clin Immunol. 2019;19(3):229–35. https://doi.org/10.1097/ACI.0000000000000523.

27. Macdougall JD, Thomas KO, Iweala OI. The meat of the matter: understanding and managing alpha-gal syndrome. Immuno Targets Ther. 2022;11:37–54. https://doi.org/10.2147/ITT.S276872.
28. Wilson JM, Schuyler AJ, Workman L, Gupta M, James HR, Posthumus J, et al. Investigation into the α-Gal syndrome: characteristics of 261 children and adults reporting red meat allergy. J Allergy Clin Immunol Pract. 2019;7(7):2348–58.e4. https://doi.org/10.1016/j.jaip.2019.03.031.
29. Carson AS, Gardner A, Iweala OI. Where's the beef?: understanding allergic responses to red meat in alpha-gal syndrome. J Immunol. 2022;208(2):267–77. https://doi.org/10.4049/jimmunol.2100712.

Index

M. G. Múnera Gómez et al. (eds.), *Allergies, Poisoning and Intolerance to Common Substances*, https://doi.org/10.1007/978-3-031-93658-6

MIX
Papier aus verantwortungsvollen Quellen
Paper from responsible sources
FSC® C105338

If you have any concerns about our products,
you can contact us on
ProductSafety@springernature.com

In case Publisher is established outside the EU,
the EU authorized representative is:
Springer Nature Customer Service Center GmbH
Europaplatz 3, 69115 Heidelberg, Germany

Printed by Libri Plureos GmbH
in Hamburg, Germany